Differential Diagnosis
of Movement Disorders
in Clinical Practice

T0211656

Abdul Qayyum Rana • Peter Hedera

Differential Diagnosis of Movement Disorders in Clinical Practice

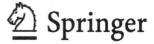 Springer

Abdul Qayyum Rana
Parkinson's Clinic
of Eastern Toronto
Toronto, ON
Canada

Peter Hedera
Department of Neurology
Division of Movement
Disorders
Vanderbilt University
Nashville, TN
USA

ISBN 978-3-319-01606-1   ISBN 978-3-319-01607-8   (eBook)
DOI 10.1007/978-3-319-01607-8
Springer Cham Heidelberg New York Dordrecht London

Library of Congress Control Number: 2013950487

Printed on acid-free paper

Springer is part of Springer Science+Business Media (www.springer.com)

Preface

Movement disorders are neurological conditions characterized by excessive involuntary movements or paucity of normal movements. Movement disorders may be complex, and thus diagnosing them can be a challenge at times. Movement disorders have wide phenomenology and have been known in human history for long time since they attract visual attention. Although some patients could have multiple types of movements, most patients present with one dominant type of abnormal movement.

We have been students of movement disorders for several years and have realized that recognizing the abnormal movement and classifying it makes the basis of differential diagnosis. Thus, closely observing the abnormal movement is very important. There are five common types of movements which patients may present with in a neurology clinic. Therefore, this handbook has been divided into five chapters. Each chapter begins with the definition of abnormal movement, and then classification, investigations, and other relevant information are given. This is followed by a brief discussion of commonly associated neurological conditions in which the given phenomenology is seen. Since this guide discusses the etiology, pathophysiology, symptoms, and treatments of these conditions only briefly, readers are encouraged to use other textbooks if the content of this manual is found insufficient.

This guide may be used by medical students, general practitioners, and other healthcare professionals. The information in this manual has been simplified to a great extent. Some of the information in this guide may represent an overview of the work of many experts in this field. Every effort has been made to present correct and up-to-date information in this handbook, but medicine is a field with ongoing research and developments; therefore, readers should refer to other sources for latest information.

Most of the information presented in this manual is considered generally accepted practice; however, the author and the publisher are not responsible for any errors, omissions, or consequences from the application of this information and make no expressed or implied warranty of the accuracy of the contents of this publication. The reader is advised to check the package insert of each drug for its indications, dosage, and warnings. Some of the information in this booklet is based upon the author's personal observation and may not be in accordance with the experience of the experts in this field.

Toronto, ON, Canada   Abdul Qayyum Rana
Nashville, TN, USA   Peter Hedera

Contents

Chapter 1
Tremor

Abstract Tremor is the most common abnormal movement and is defined as an involuntary, rhythmic oscillation of a body part. This chapter reviews main characteristics of tremor, such as body segments affected by tremor (arm, head vocal cords), segment position when tremor is observed (resting and action tremor), frequency and amplitude of tremor. The main emphasis is on the most common causes of tremor, essential tremor and Parkinson's disease. We discuss main clinical features of tremor seen with these two common neurologic problems, their differential diagnosis, and main therapeutic options. Additionally, other less common causes of tremor are also briefly discussed.

Keywords Tremor • Therapy • Essential tremor • Parkinson's disease • Deep brain stimulation

1.1 Introduction

Tremor is defined as an involuntary, rhythmic oscillation of a body part. Tremor is the most commonly seen abnormal movement among all of the movement disorders. Essential tremor is the most common movement disorder. Tremor can be of many different types as follows:

A.Q. Rana, P. Hedera, *Differential Diagnosis of Movement Disorders in Clinical Practice*, DOI 10.1007/978-3-319-01607-8_1,
© Springer International Publishing Switzerland 2014

I. *Resting tremor*

A resting tremor usually manifests itself when the affected body part is not voluntarily activated and is in a state of completed relaxation supported against gravity. The resting tremor either diminishes or completely disappears during the onset of voluntary activity. Some of the common causes of resting tremor are as follows:

(a) Parkinson's disease.
(b) Parkinson plus syndromes.
(c) Midbrain tremor (Holmes tremor).
(d) Wilson's disease.
(e) Essential tremor, when severe, may have a resting component, and resting tremor can be seen in about 10–15 % of patients with essential tremor. Patients with essential tremor typically do not manifest resting tremor while walking, and this may be a useful feature to distinguish it from resting tremor in Parkinson's disease, which persists during gait.

II. *Action tremor*

An action tremor occurs during voluntary activity of the affected body part or when the affected body part is maintaining a steady posture against gravity and either diminishes or completely disappears at rest. This includes postural and kinetic tremors.

A postural tremor occurs when the affected body part is voluntarily maintaining a position against gravity. True postural tremor appears without any time delay, and it needs to be distinguished from a reemergent tremor, which is observed after 5–20 s and represents resting tremor.

A kinetic tremor occurs when the affected body part is performing a voluntary activity which could be goal directed or non-goal directed.

Some examples of action tremor are:

(a) Essential tremor
(b) Primary writing tremor

(c) Enhanced physiological tremor:

    (i) Emotional stress or anxiety

    (ii) Endocrine: thyrotoxicosis, hypoglycemia, adreno-corticosteroids, and pheochromocytoma

(d) Cerebellar tremor

(e) Drug- and toxin-induced tremor such as beta agonists, lithium, neuroleptics, theophylline, valproic acid, lead, mercury, manganese, and arsenic

(f) Peripheral neuropathy

III. *Intention tremor*
An intention tremor is present if the amplitude of the tremor increases when the affected body part is approaching the target. Intention tremor is seen in cerebellar pathology.

IV. *Task-specific kinetic tremor*
A task-specific kinetic tremor occurs during a specific activity, such as primary writing tremor.

1.1.1 Classification

According to Position of the Body Part Affected by Tremor

Tremor is categorized as resting tremor (if the tremor occurs while the affected body part is in complete repose), postural tremor (if the tremor occurs while the affected body part is in steady posture), or kinetic tremor (if the tremor occurs while the affected body part is exerting a movement).

According to the Regions of Body Affected

Tremor may affect different body parts including the limbs, head, tongue, jaw, vocal cords, and palate. The parts of the body that are affected by tremor depend upon the underlying neurological condition.

According to the Frequency of Tremor

1. Low-frequency tremor, e.g., tremor of Parkinson's disease
2. Medium-frequency tremor, e.g., essential tremor
3. High-frequency tremor, e.g., orthostatic tremor

According to the Amplitude of Tremor

1. Mild amplitude
2. Moderate amplitude
3. Severe amplitude

According to the Etiology of Tremor

1. Essential tremor.
2. Enhanced physiological tremor.
3. Drug- or toxin-induced tremor.
4. Dystonic tremor.
5. Cerebellar tremor.
6. Holmes tremor (midbrain tremor).
7. Primary orthostatic tremor.
8. Cortical tremor.
9. Peripheral neuropathy-associated tremor.
10. Tremor of Parkinson's disease.
11. Psychogenic tremor.
12. Tremor is also seen in many other medical conditions such as thyroid disease, Wilson's disease, hypoxia, hypotension, AIDS, and hereditary hemochromatosis.
13. Task-specific tremor such as primary writing tremor.
14. Posttraumatic tremor.

As previously mentioned, essential tremor is the most common movement disorder.

1.1.2   Description

The following parameters should be taken into account when describing a particular tremor:

TABLE 1.1 Approximate frequencies of various tremor syndromes

Tremor syndrome	Frequency (Hz)
Enhanced physiological tremor	10–14
Essential tremor syndrome	7–10
Primary orthostatic tremor	14–18
Task-specific tremor	4–8
Holmes tremor	3–5
Tremor of Parkinson's disease	3–7
Cerebellar tremor	3–5
Palatal tremor	2–6
Dystonic tremor	5–7
Alcoholic tremor	3–4
Toxic- and drug-induced tremor	5–10
Psychogenic tremor	Variable

1. The affected body part. Also known as topography (e.g., head, limbs, chin, jaw)
2. The frequency of the tremor
3. The position of affected body part in which tremor is most prominent (e.g., rest, postural, activity, specific task)
4. The amplitude of tremor

1.2 Frequencies of Various Tremor Syndromes

Different tremor syndromes have different frequencies. Approximate frequencies of various tremor syndromes are described in Table 1.1.

1.2.1 Investigations

In most cases of tremor, no investigations are necessary. However, when other alternative conditions are suspected, the investigations may be directed to the possible underlying cause.

Investigations including thyroid function tests and brain imaging such as CT scan or MRI of brain may be required in some cases, especially if any cerebellar or focal long tract signs are present. In patients with suspicion of Wilson's disease, 24 h urine copper, serum ceruloplasmin, and copper as well as slit lamp examination for Kayser-Fleischer rings may be performed for initial assessment.

1.2.2   Causes

Essential tremor
Enhanced physiological tremor
Tremor of Parkinson's disease
Dystonic tremor
Task-specific tremor such as primary writing tremor
Cerebellar tremor
Drug- or toxin-induced tremor
Holmes tremor (midbrain tremor)
Primary orthostatic tremor
Alcohol induced tremor
Cortical tremor
Peripheral neuropathy-associated tremor
Psychogenic tremor
Tremor associated with medical conditions such as thyroid
    disease, Wilson's disease, hypoxia, hypotension, AIDS, and
    hereditary hemochromatosis
Posttraumatic tremor

1.3   Essential Tremor

Essential tremor affects 5–6 % of the patients over the age of 65. About 5–15 % of essential tremor cases occur during childhood. Essential tremor may be familial in 50–60 % of all cases and typically starts before the age of 65 years. Essential tremor is common in all races across the world.

The prevalence of essential tremor is significantly higher in individuals above the age of 40. In some studies, the prevalence of essential tremor in patients above the age of 40 has been reported to be as high as 10 %; however, the peak age of onset for essential tremor is 70–79 years. The prevalence of essential tremor is ten times greater in 70- to 79-year-old individuals as compared to 40- to 69-year-old individuals. Some studies have reported a slightly higher prevalence in men, but other studies could not find any difference between men and women.

The likelihood of patients with essential tremor having first-degree relatives with essential tremor is five times greater than the normal population. There seems to be an increase in prevalence of essential tremor with age. It is estimated that almost five million people in the USA, over the age of 40, are affected with essential tremor. Essential tremor is more common than Parkinson's disease.

Essential tremor usually affects both sides of the body, although initially it may only be noticed on one side and up to 15 % of ET patients may have strictly unilateral tremor. It can occur at any age. Although, it may be seen in the early 20s, late onset, after the age of 55 years is more common. Essential tremor may begin in early childhood, but its prevalence and intensity increase with advancing age, and eventually, it may interfere with writing, eating, and other activities of daily life. In familial cases, the onset of essential tremor may be much earlier than sporadic cases.

Essential tremor is a slowly progressive condition in which the amplitude of tremor usually increases with time. In some cases there may be no change noted in the tremor for several years, and then in advanced age, the tremor may get worse relatively quickly. In addition, as the amplitude of tremor increases, the frequency of tremor may decrease.

Fatigue, central nervous system stimulation, sexual arousal, emotional excitement, and temperature extremes can exacerbate the tremor. Alcohol may dampen the tremor significantly. The history of response to alcohol is helpful diagnostically. The effect of alcohol seems to be centrally mediated. Caffeine, on the other hand, seems to precipitate essential tremor. Essential tremor, like most other movement disorders, disappears in sleep.

1.3.1   Etiology and Pathogenesis

The exact cause of essential tremor is unknown. Some patients may have a family history of tremor in their parents, siblings, or close relatives. However, sporadic cases are seen quite frequently. The exact mechanism of inheritance is unclear. In a significant number of cases, essential tremor is hereditary and is transmitted in an autosomal dominant pattern. Chromosomes 3q13, 2p22–p25, and 6p23 have been suggested to be the disease loci in many reports. More recently, common sequence variants in *LINGO1* have been suggested a risk factor for ET. Environmental factors may also play a role in the causation of essential tremor. This is supported by the lack of a complete concordance of essential tremor in monozygotic twins.

There is a lack of clear understanding of the pathophysiological mechanisms of essential tremor. The central nervous system pathology is supported by the observation of response of tremor to thalamotomy and centrally acting drugs. Cerebellum may play an important role in pathophysiology of essential tremor. It is believed that essential tremor may emerge from abnormal oscillations within thalamocortical and cerebello-olivary loops in the brain. This theory is supported by the findings that the lesions or injury of the cerebellar and thalamic regions reduces the intensity of essential tremor. Neuronal discharges correlated to tremor have been observed to occur in the ventrolateral thalamus, particularly in the ventralis intermedius nucleus. Contralateral limb tremor can be suppressed by the ablation or high-frequency stimulation of ventralis intermedius nucleus of the thalamus. Essential tremor may be the result of abnormal oscillations of a central nervous system pacemaker. This central oscillator could be enhanced or suppressed; however, the exact location of this oscillator is unknown. Another theory considers ET a neurodegenerative disorders with a selective degeneration of Purkinje cerebellar cells.

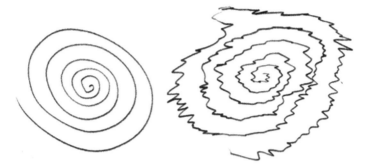

FIGURE 1.1   Spiral drawing by the examiner and a patient with essential tremor (spiral test)

1.3.2   Clinical Features

Patients usually complain of their handwriting becoming sloppy, large, and irregular; trouble holding objects like a cup full of liquid; and trouble using a fork, spoon, keys, and screwdriver, pouring liquids, and shaving (Fig. 1.1). They may spill liquids and writing a check may be a challenge. In severe cases essential tremor can interfere with dressing, preparing meals, and other activities of daily living.

The pediatric cases of essential tremor affect more males than females. Most patients with essential tremor seek attention only if they have a functional or social disability because of tremor. Essential tremor may result in social phobia due to embarrassment.

Patients with essential tremor may have mild neuropsychological deficits, including problems with visual perception, encoding, and verbal fluency as well as working memory.

Classical essential tremor is a monosymptomatic, postural, and action tremor. Essential tremor usually affects the upper extremities and the hands, but it may also involve the head, lower extremities, voice, and other body parts. In classic essential tremor, the approximate frequency of involvement of different body parts is summarized in Table 1.2.

TABLE 1.2 Approximate frequency of involvement of different body regions in essential tremor

Region of body	Frequency (%)
Hands and arms	90
Head	30
Legs	25–30
Voice	10–15
Trunk	5
Face	5
Tongue	4

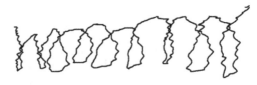

FIGURE 1.2 Multiple loops drawing in a patient with essential tremor

1.3.3   Characteristics of Essential Tremor

Essential tremor is only present when the affected body part is exerting effort and not during repose. Mental tasks or stress may exacerbate the essential tremor. Essential tremor does not occur during sleep, but patients sometimes complain of an especially coarse tremor upon awakening in the morning.

Essential tremor affecting the hands causes a flexion extension movement of the hands, abduction movement of the fingers, and, only in minority of cases, supination-pronation movements of the hands or arms. The size of handwriting is usually large (macrographia) in contrast to the tremor of Parkinson's disease, in which the size of handwriting is small (micrographia) (Fig. 1.2). The legs, tongue, voice, face, and trunk, if involved in essential tremor, are usually affected in the later stages of the disease.

The tremor of the hands is usually of medium frequency in the range of 7–10 Hz. It becomes more apparent with arms outstretched, extended, or straight at elbows with fingers apart, as well as with arms outstretched, flexed at elbows in front of the chest with fingers apart (wing-beating position), and during the finger-nose-finger movements.

The frequency of tremor varies with age, severity, and the location in the body. The tremor frequency usually slows down with age, at a rate of about 0.07 Hz/year. This decrease in frequency causes a gradual increase in tremor amplitude over the years. Patients with severe essential tremor may also have difficulty with tandem gait, which is tested by walking heel to toe. Neurological examination is otherwise normal. Essential tremor in the upper limbs is usually symmetric or only mildly asymmetric.

1.3.4 Diagnosis of Essential Tremor

The diagnosis of essential tremor is made by history and physical examination. The following steps are helpful in the assessment of essential tremor:

1. Asking the patient to hold arms straight outstretched, extended at elbows with fingers spread apart.
2. Holding arms with fingers outstretched, flexed at elbows in front of the chest (wing-beating position).
3. While arms in the wing-beating position, asking the patients to make a fist of both hands except leaving their index finger of each hand extended pointing across each other in close proximity without touching (also known as one-to-one test). This helps to assess the subtle cases of postural tremor.
4. Finger-nose-finger testing.
5. Asking the patient to hold a cup full of water and to bring it to their lips and then away from their mouth a few times to see if there is any spillage of water (glass test). Pouring of liquids may also be tested.
6. Writing a standard sentence on each visit (Fig. 1.3). The new writing sample on each visit is then compared to the

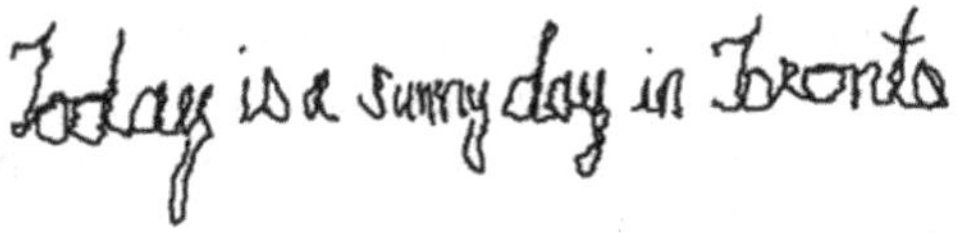

FIGURE 1.3 Handwriting of a patient with very mild essential tremor

writing sample from the previous visit in order to assess the therapeutic response.

7. Drawing a spiral without supporting the hand on the clipboard on each visit and comparing the drawing to the one from previous visit in order to assess the therapeutic response.

8. Examination of voice by holding a prolonged note; head, tongue, and heel-knee-shin testing; and tandem gait are important parts of assessment of essential tremor.

In typical cases of essential tremor, no investigations are required. When considering the diagnosis of essential tremor, the primary inclusion features are as follows:

1. Postural or kinetic tremor of both upper extremities
2. Isolated head tremor without any dystonic features
3. Absence of other focal findings except mild cogwheeling, especially in the elderly patients

1.3.5 Treatment of Essential Tremor

Medicinal Treatment

Sometimes patients with essential tremor may desire nothing more than to be assured that they do not have Parkinson's disease. Any exacerbating factors, if present, should be addressed first. The avoidance of stimulants, such as caffeine, is helpful in some cases. If the tremor does not affect daily functioning, it could be observed. Milder cases of essential tremor may be helped with occupational therapy training or use of weighted wrist bracelets that are available at many sports stores.

Alcohol may transiently reduce tremor amplitude in about 50–90 % of the cases, but the rebound tremor may be worse when the effect of alcohol wears off. Alcohol intake is not recommended for treatment of essential tremor.

The most commonly used medications are propranolol, a beta-blocker, and primidone, a GABA agonist (Table 1.3).

Beta-Blockers

Among the beta-blockers, the most effective medication is *propranolol*. Drugs that are predominantly *B-1* antagonists are less effective than those that act on *B-2* receptors as well. Overall, about 25 % of patients are able to maintain their initial improvement for about 2 years. It is a nonselective beta-adrenergic receptor antagonist. Some patients may take propranolol only before social engagements, whereas others may use it on a daily basis. If propranolol is to be taken on daily basis, the dosage ranges from 60 to 260 mg/day. Propranolol is effective in treating essential tremor involving limbs, and many studies have shown that the magnitude of tremor is reduced by at least 50 % as measured by accelerometry and clinical rating scale.

Side effects include a drop in blood pressure, fatigue, depression, impotence, and bradycardia. Propranolol is contraindicated in patients with asthma, COPD, or heart failure. Diabetes mellitus is also a relative contraindication as propranolol can mask symptoms of hypoglycemia.

Propranolol LA may be taken only once a day as it is a long-acting preparation. Propranolol LA is also effective in improving limb tremor. In one study propranolol LA caused about 30–38 % improvement in limb tremor when measured by accelerometry. Propranolol, propranolol LA, and primidone exhibit a similar therapeutic effect for the limb tremor.

Atenolol also has a positive therapeutic effect on limb tremor. The dose is 50–150 mg/day. About 25 % mean improvement on the clinical rating scale and a 37 % improvement by accelerometry were noticed in one study. However, side effects such as lightheadedness, nausea, cough, dry mouth, and sleepiness may limit its use.

TABLE 1.3 Pharmacological agents used in the treatment of essential tremor

Drug	Dose	Side effects	Comments
Primidone	Starting dose is 31.25 mg HS, increased slowly up to 250 mg TID	Sedation, drowsiness, fatigue, nausea, vomiting, malaise, and dizziness	GABA agonist
Propranolol	Starting dose is 40 mg BID, increased slowly up to 180 mg BID	Postural hypotension, bradycardia, drowsiness, impotence, fatigue, depression	B1/B2 antagonist
Topiramate	Starting dose is 25 mg Hs, increased weekly by 50 mg/day to the maximum dose of 200 mg BID	Weight loss, tingling and paresthesias, concentration difficulties, exacerbation of glaucoma, and renal stones	Sodium channel blocker
Gabapentin	Starting dose is 300 mg HS, increased over few days to 300–900 mg TID	Fatigue, dizziness, nervousness, lethargy	Alpha-2-delta calcium channel subunit blocker
Nadolol	Starting dose is 40 mg once daily, maximum 240 mg/day	Dizziness	B1/B2 antagonist
Atenolol	Starting dose is 50 mg once daily, maximum150 mg/day	Postural hypotension, lightheadedness, nausea, cough, dry mouth, sleepiness	B1 antagonist
Clonazepam	Starting dose is 0.5 mg TID to 2 mg/day	Lethargy	Benzodiazepine
Botulinum toxin A for head tremor	Dose ranges from 50 to 400 units depending upon muscles involved and degree of tremor	Excessive weakness of injected muscles, dysphagia, injection pain	Injected every 3–4 months

In one study, *nadolol*, at a dose of 120–240 mg daily, resulted in about 60–70 % improvement by accelerometry in patients who previously responded to propranolol. The side effects include dizziness.

Primidone

Primidone, conventionally used as an antiepileptic medication, provides a significant therapeutic benefit for essential tremor. It is a GABA agonist. The initial dose is one quarter of a tablet of 125 mg (31.25 mg) which is increased slowly. The average reduction in tremor is at least 50 % when measured by the clinical rating scale and accelerometry. One third of the patients may have a strong feeling of being unwell and experience side effects of drowsiness, confusion, nausea, and dizziness upon the initiation of this drug. However, these side effects may improve in 2–3 weeks time.

Combined treatment with propranolol and primidone may be more effective than monotherapy with either of these agents alone. In one study, the addition of 50–1,000 mg/day of primidone to propranolol reduced the tremor amplitude more than when propranolol was used alone. Propranolol at an average dosage of 260 mg/day (its maximum effective dosage) reduced tremor amplitude by a mean of 35 %, but the addition of primidone (50–1,000 mg/day) decreased the tremor amplitude by a mean of 60–70 %.

Propranolol and primidone alone are almost equally effective in the treatment of both postural and kinetic tremor, but the combination of these two drugs is more effective than either drug used alone. The combined treatment with primidone and propranolol can be used to treat limb tremor when monotherapy is not sufficient. The therapeutic effects of primidone and propranolol on postural and kinetic tremor last for at least several years. However, the response may decrease partially with time. The dosage of primidone and propranolol may need to be increased with time.

Other Therapies

Topiramate is a sodium channel blocker. Its common indications include epilepsy and prophylaxis of migraine. It has a mild to moderate effect in reducing essential tremor. In one study, it resulted in about a 22–37 % mean improvement in limb tremor when measured by the clinical rating scale. The initial starting dose of topiramate is 25 mg once a day, a dosage which is increased slowly to two or three times daily. Side effects include decrease in appetite, weight loss, paresthesias, concentration difficulties, exacerbation of glaucoma, and renal stone.

Gabapentin has a mild to moderate beneficial effect on essential tremor. In one study, gabapentin reduced postural and kinetic tremor when administered at a dose of 1,200 mg/day. When gabapentin was used as a monotherapy, there was about a 77 % improvement by accelerometry and a 33 % improvement on the clinical rating scale. The side effects include fatigue, dizziness, nervousness, and lethargy.

Pregabalin has a similar efficacy as gabapentin, and initial doses at 50 mg/day with the maximum dose of 600 mg/day reduce tremor severity at the mean dose of 286 mg/day. Side effects profile is very similar to gabapentin.

In one study, benzodiazepines, especially *clonazepam*, significantly reduced the kinetic tremor. There was about a 71 % mean improvement by accelerometry and a 26–57 % improvement in limb tremor on the clinical rating scale. The dose ranged from 0.5 to 6 mg/day. Side effects include drowsiness. There is a potential of abuse and possibility of withdrawal symptoms associated with clonazepam, and therefore it should be used with a great caution.

Treatment of limb tremor with atenolol, topiramate, and gabapentin is not as effective as propranolol or primidone. Therefore, atenolol, topiramate, and gabapentin are considered for treatment of postural and kinetic limb tremor if propranolol or primidone are not helpful.

Botulinum toxin may offer some improvement but may cause finger or wrist weakness. Botulinum toxin has been used to treat hand, head, and voice tremor variants of the essential tremor syndrome. About a 67 % improvement in head tremor was noticed by accelerometry in one study. The side effects include pain at the injection site and weakness. The effect of botulinum toxin on essential tremor affecting limbs is mild. About a 20 % improvement in postural tremor and a 27 % improvement in kinetic tremor were noticed in one study. It may reduce head and voice tremor, but when used to treat voice tremor, botulinum toxin may cause hoarseness of voice and swallowing difficulties. In one study, about a 22 % improvement with unilateral injections and a 30 % improvement with bilateral injections were noticed in voice tremor. The botulinum toxin injections for limb, head, and voice tremor may be considered in medically refractory cases.

Surgical Treatments

Surgical treatments are used for patients who have very advanced essential tremor which is refractory to the pharmacological management. Two types of surgical treatments are done: *thalamotomy* and *deep brain thalamic stimulation* (Table 1.4).

Surgical procedures such as stimulation of the nucleus ventralis intermedius or ablation are used for intractable tremor, and a significant improvement in the tremor has been reported. In presurgical assessment, patients are evaluated by a multidisciplinary team, including a neurologist with expertise in movement disorders, a neurosurgeon, and a neuropsychologist. Appropriate brain imaging is also performed. The procedure may be unilateral or bilateral depending on the degree of tremor.

1. *Unilateral deep brain stimulation* results in marked improvement of contralateral postural and kinetic tremor. In one study, about a 60–90 % improvement on the clinical rating scale was noticed in limb tremor. Voice tremor usually does not improve by the unilateral nucleus ventralis intermedius stimulation. Inconsistent results have been reported about the response of head tremor to unilateral or bilateral deep brain stimulation. Deep brain stimulation has shown greater improvement and fewer side effects than thalamotomy. However, these procedures are invasive, and side effects like speech and swallowing problems, sensory disturbances, and

TABLE 1.4 Surgical treatments of essential tremor

Technique	Side effects	Comments
Thalamotomy	Transient contralateral weakness, dysarthria, contralateral hemiparesis, verbal or cognitive deficits, and confusion	Marked improvement of contralateral tremor. Side effects are much more pronounced with bilateral procedure, and bilateral thalamotomy is not recommended
Gamma knife thalamotomy	Transient contralateral arm weakness and numbness, dysarthria, dystonia of the contralateral arm and leg	Insufficient evidence. May be similar to thalamotomy and only unilateral procedure is performed
Deep brain thalamic stimulation	Dysarthria, weakness, numbness, headache, intracranial hemorrhage, disequilibrium, and decreased verbal fluency	Marked improvement in limb tremor, insufficient evidence for voice and head tremors. Side effects less than in thalamotomy and include dysesthesia and dysarthria. Bilateral procedure is commonly performed if indicated

balance problems may occur. There is also a risk of infection and hemorrhage associated with these procedures. The side effects of this treatment can usually be reduced by adjusting the stimulus parameters, but this may result in reduced tremor suppression and efficacy.

2. *Unilateral thalamotomy* is very effective for the treatment of contralateral limb tremor, while bilateral thalamotomy has frequent and severe side effects. In one study, about a 55–90 % improvement on the clinical rating scale was noticed. Relief of essential tremor after thalamotomy has been thought to be related to disruption of abnormal thalamocortical synchronization. The first thalamotomy for essential tremor was performed in the early 1960s.

3. *Gamma knife thalamotomy* is performed by delivering radiation to an intracranial target determined by brain imaging. In

one study, there was about a 70–80 % improvement seen on the clinical rating scale; however, some delayed complications have been reported with this technique. Although good results have been reported in several studies, the evidence is insufficient to recommend this treatment for essential tremor.

Focused ultrasound is another method for lesioning of ViM, but its wider use requires further safety and outcome studies.

Prognosis of essential tremor is a lifelong disorder that gradually worsens with advancing age. The life span and the general health of the patient are not affected. This condition causes significant interference with employment, daily activities, and social functioning.

1.4 Enhanced Physiological Tremor

Enhanced physiological tremor is a result of the interaction of numerous mechanical and neuromuscular influences. This type of tremor can be enhanced in amplitude by various psychological and metabolic aggravating factors which include anxiety, fatigue, alcohol withdrawal, and hyperthyroidism. Caffeine can also enhance this type of tremor. This tremor has a frequency of 10–14 Hz. Some patients with ET may initially experience tremor consistent with enhanced physiologic tremor before developing more typical constant tremor.

1.5 Parkinson's Disease

Parkinson's disease is a neurodegenerative condition initially described by James Parkinson in 1817. Parkinson's disease has an approximate incidence of 20/100,000 and prevalence of 160/100,000. PD makes up about 80 % of cases of parkinsonism. The exact cause of Parkinson's disease is unknown. About 90 % of cases are sporadic. There are definite genetic causes of PD in about 10 % of cases. The current hypothesis is that Parkinson's disease may result from interaction between environmental factors and genetic susceptibility.

Parkinson's disease arises from loss of dopaminergic neurons mainly in substantia nigra pars compacta of midbrain. The neurodegenerative changes are not restricted to nigrostriatal pathway however and involve many other dopaminergic and non-dopaminergic cell groups such as locus coeruleus, nucleus basalis of Meynert, and raphe nuclei which may underlie nonmotor symptoms and cognitive dysfunction in Parkinson's disease. Parkinson's disease causes both motor and nonmotor symptoms.

Motor symptoms of Parkinson's disease include bradykinesia, rigidity, resting tremor, and postural instability. *Parkinson's disease tremor* is classically a resting tremor that is present when the affected body part is in repose and diminishes with activity and posture. The frequency of the tremor of Parkinson's disease is low, in the range of 3–7 Hz (Table 1.5). It is usually of supination-pronation type and starts on one side of the body, mostly in the hand or arm. It is also referred as pill-rolling tremor when it involves the thumb and index finger. The resting tremor of Parkinson's disease typically starts asymmetrically in the thumb or index finger and involves the hands, arms, legs, and lips but usually does not involve the head or voice. This type of tremor is usually accompanied by other signs of Parkinson's disease such as bradykinesia and rigidity. Postural instability is usually not seen in the early stages of Parkinson's disease. History of the other features of Parkinson's disease such as difficulty with dexterity and micrographia may also be elicited (Fig. 1.4).

About 40 % of the patients with Parkinson's disease may have postural and action tremor in addition to the typical resting tremor of Parkinson's disease. Postural and action tremor may occur in isolation or in combination with resting tremor in Parkinson's disease. In the face, resting tremor actually affects the lips and jaw, and the patient may notice a rhythmic clicking of the teeth.

The prominent head tremor is rarely caused by Parkinson's disease. The severe limb tremor of Parkinson's disease may be conducted to the trunk and head. The tremor in the legs, especially in the feet, while sitting is usually due to Parkinson's

TABLE 1.5 Comparison of enhanced physiological, essential, and Parkinson's disease tremor

	Enhanced physiological tremor	Essential tremor	Tremor of Parkinson's disease
Body part affected	Hands	Hands, head, voice	Hands or arms > legs
Accompanying symptoms	None or symptoms of anxiety state	None	Rigidity, bradykinesia, and postural instability
Frequency	10–14 Hz	7–10 Hz	3–7 Hz
Positional component	Posture > kinetic	Posture > kinetic, may have a slight resting component if severe	Resting, may have a postural and kinetic component in severe cases
Symmetry	Bilateral, symmetric	Bilateral, can be mildly asymmetrical	Initially unilateral, bilateral, and symmetrical in advanced stage
Course	Usually nonprogressive	Progressive	Progressive
Response to alcohol	Minimal or none	Responds significantly	None
Effect of caffeine, stress, stimulants	Increases	May increase	Increases with mental tasks
Inheritance	None	Autosomal dominant with variable penetrance	Sporadic or related to genetics of Parkinson's disease

disease. Essential tremor usually appears without any latency when the arms are outstretched, while the tremor of Parkinson's disease appears after a latency of at least several

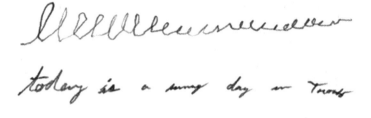

FIGURE 1.4 Multiple loops and handwriting of a patient with tremor of Parkinson's disease with worsening of micrographia

seconds when the arms are outstretched from the resting position (reemergent tremor). About 20–30 % of patients with Parkinson's disease may not have tremor.

Bradykinesia is a cardinal and most disabling feature Parkinson's disease. It has various manifestations such as slowness of movement while performing activities of daily life (ADLs). Patients may also experience difficulty fastening buttons, cutting food, or tying shoelaces.

Rigidity is present in limbs and may or may not be present in neck (limbs more than neck in idiopathic Parkinson's disease). Posture is typically stooped (Fig. 1.5). However, balance problems and postural instability are usually seen in moderate to advanced stages of Parkinson's disease. It is also a very disabling symptom may not respond to medications and may lead to falls.

1.5.1   Etiology and Pathophysiology of Parkinson's Disease

Exact etiology of Parkinson's disease is unknown. Parkinson's disease has sporadic and genetic causes. The current hypothesis is that Parkinson's disease may result from interaction between environmental factors and genetic susceptibility. About 90 % of cases of PD are sporadic without any genetic linkage, but there are definite genetic cases of PD.

Parkinson's disease involves loss of dopaminergic neurons mainly in substantia nigra pars compacta of midbrain. The main pathological feature of Parkinson's disease is the loss of

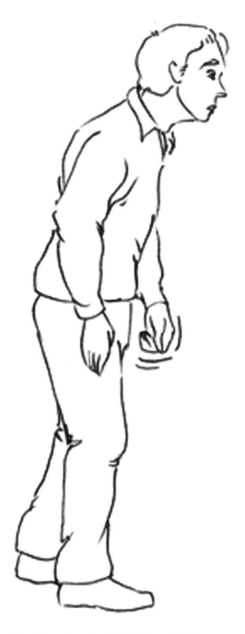

FIGURE 1.5 Stooping of posture in Parkinson's disease

neuromelanin-containing dopaminergic neurons of nigrostriatal pathway resulting in depletion of dopamine which leads
to motor symptoms such as bradykinesia, rigidity, resting
tremor, and postural instability. The degenerative changes in
Parkinson's disease are not restricted to nigrostriatal pathway
and involve many other dopaminergic and non-dopaminergic
cell groups such as the locus coeruleus, nucleus basalis of
Meynert, and raphe nuclei which may be the cause of nonmotor symptoms Parkinson's disease. Lewy bodies are eosino-
philic spherical cytoplasmic fibrillary aggregates composed of
a variety of proteins including alpha-synuclein, ubiquitin, and
parkin and are the hallmark of Parkinson's disease.

1.5.2   Nonmotor Symptoms of Parkinson's Disease

Parkinson's disease also causes many nonmotor symptoms
such as cognitive dysfunction, depression, anxiety, visual hallucinations, sleep disturbances, reduced facial expression,
drooling, speech problems, and autonomic disturbances
including urinary and sexual dysfunction, postural hypotension, constipation, decreased sense of smell, decreased sense
of taste, and difficulty swallowing. Several nonmotor symptoms, such as REM sleep behavior or anxiety, may actually
precede the onset of motor symptoms.

More than one third of patients with Parkinson's disease
develop cognitive dysfunction which includes impaired executive and visuospatial functioning. There may also be impairment of attention, but memory and language may remain
intact. Treatment of cognitive dysfunction includes cholines-
terase inhibitors such as rivastigmine or donepezil. Memantine
may provide additional benefit.

About 40 % of patients may have depression sometimes
in the course of Parkinson's disease. Mechanism of depression may involve deficiency of multiple neurotransmitters in
mesocortical monoaminergic systems, including dopaminergic projections, noradrenergic, and serotoninergic projections.

Commonly used treatment includes selective serotonin reuptake inhibitors such as paroxetine, sertraline, or fluvoxamine.

Sleep disturbances affect more than two thirds of patients with Parkinson's disease and include multiple awakenings with difficulty falling asleep, insomnia, excessive daytime sleepiness (EDS), and REM sleep behavioral disorder. Principals of sleep hygiene may be helpful. Benzodiazepines may be helpful to suppress REM phase of sleep and reduce manifestations of REM sleep behavior, which is consistent with "acting of dreams." Melatonin may be also helpful for this problem. The emergence of REM sleep behavior in patients with manifesting motor problems increases the risk of cognitive decline.

Speech disorders occur in about 80–90 % of PD patients as the disease progresses and include softening of voice (hypophonia), difficulty in initiation of speech (start hesitation of speech), low volume of voice, monotonous speech, fast and slurred of speech, and decrease of the content of spontaneous speech. Speech therapy is helpful to improve communication skills. Lee Silverman Voice Training (LSVT) and Pitch Limiting Voice Training (PLVT) programs are used by many speech pathologists.

Swallowing dysfunction may be present in nearly half of the Parkinson's disease patients, and consultations with a speech pathologist are usually required. Constipation is reported by more than 90 % of patients with Parkinson's disease. There is an early involvement of both extrinsic and intrinsic innervations of the gut with Lewy body pathology in Parkinson's disease.

Urinary dysfunction is reported by 37–70 % of Parkinson's disease patients. The common symptoms of urinary dysfunction include urgency or increased frequency of urination and nocturia. Urinary dysfunction does not occur in the beginning of the course of PD. If the patients have urinary dysfunction in the beginning of the course of Parkinson's disease, atypical parkinsonism such as MSA may be considered in the differential diagnosis. Urinary bladder dysfunction is caused by detrusor muscle hyperreflexia, whereas detrusor hypoactivity is less common. Also paradoxical cocontraction of urethral sphincter muscle has been described as an OFF-period phenomenon. Medications such as tolterodine (Detrol LA®) are generally considered to be useful; however, anticholinergic side effects could occur especially in the elderly.

Sexual dysfunction affects at least one third of patients with Parkinson's disease. Autonomic dysfunction is the cause of erectile failure in men. Women may have decreased libido and orgasm. Sexual dysfunction usually occurs in moderate to late stages of PD, and if it is present at the onset of the disease, an alternative diagnosis such as MSA should be considered. Urology consultation may be helpful.

Anxiety is usually seen in moderate to advanced stages of PD but may occur in the early stages of PD as well. Anxiety may be associated with feeling of losing control, palpitations, and dizziness, shortness of breathing, perspiration, and agitation. Cyclic anxiety may be an OFF symptom as well.

Drooling is reported by more than two thirds of Parkinson's disease patients. It is due to decreased swallowing and flexed head posture rather than hypersecretion of saliva. Initially noticed at night time only, later becomes noticeable during day time as well. Pooling of saliva in the mouth may lead to aspiration pneumonia. Scopolamine, transdermal patch (Transderm-V®), atropine 1 % drops instilled in mouth, or botulinum toxin injection is helpful.

Chronic pain is reported by two third of patients with Parkinson's disease. Some patients may report excruciating pain and sensory symptoms. These sensory symptoms mostly affect the legs, feet, and toes. Patients may report proximal limb pain as well as shoulder discomfort. Initially these symptoms may be more marked on the side that is affected most by Parkinson's disease and may be more prominent in the mornings or during the OFF period.

Postural hypotension is present in almost one third of the Parkinson's disease patients. It is usually reported as light-headedness or dizziness. Autonomic dysfunction in Parkinson's disease is the main cause of postural hypotension. Postural hypotension usually occurs in moderate to advanced stages of Parkinson's disease. Postural hypotension may result in falls and should be treated if symptomatic.

Psychosis and visual hallucinations occur in at least one third of patients with Parkinson's disease. These problems are more frequent in Parkinson's disease patients with dementia.

Parkinson's disease is diagnosed by history and neurological examination. There are no uniform criteria to diagnose Parkinson's disease. Most experts consider diagnosis of PD in the presence of bradykinesia and at least one of the signs of rigidity, resting tremor, or postural instability, in the absence of any other attributable cause or features of atypical parkinsonism.

1.5.3 Treatment of Parkinson's Disease

Pharmacological and rehabilitation treatments are the mainstay of therapy. In selected cases surgery may also be used.

1.6 Pharmacological Treatments

1. Levodopa

   (a) Levodopa/Carbidopa (*Sinemet*®)

      - Starting dose is 100/25 mg, half tablet three times daily. Levodopa provides maximum motor benefit. Side effects include nausea, lightheadedness, confusion, motor fluctuations, dyskinesia, and sleepiness.

   (b) Levodopa/Benserazide (Prolopa®)

      - Starting dose is 50/12.5 mg, to 100/25 mg three times daily; motor benefit and side effects are similar to levodopa/carbidopa.

2. *COMT Inhibitors*

   (a) Entacapone (Comtan®)
       Dosage is 200 mg in conjunction with each dose of levodopa. Side effects include urine discoloration, diarrhea, and potentiation of side effects of levodopa.
   (b) Levodopa/Carbidopa/Entacapone (Stalevo®)

This medication comes in four strengths as follows:

- 50/12.5/200
- 100/25/200
- 150/37.5/200
- 200/50/200

Side effects are similar to combination of levodopa and entacapone.

3. *Dopamine Agonists*

   (a) Pramipexole (Mirapex®)

   - Starting dose is 0.125 mg three times daily, usual maximum dose is 1.5 mg three times daily.
   - It is used in early to moderate stage of Parkinson's disease. It is avoided in elderly patients or those with cognitive dysfunction due to side effects which include sudden sleep attacks, impulse control disorders, visual hallucinations, nausea, lightheadedness, and leg edema.

   (b) Ropinirole (Requip®)

   - Starting dose is 0.25 mg three times daily, maximum dosage is 8 mg three times daily.
   - Indications and side effects are similar to pramipexole.

   (c) Rotigotine (Neupro Patch®)

   - Starting dose is 2 mg/day, maximum dose 8 mg/day.
   - Indications and side effects are similar to other dopaminergic agonists.

4. *MAOB Inhibitors*

   (a) Rasagiline (Azilect®)

   - Starting dose is 0.5 mg once daily, increased to 1 mg once daily.
   - May be used as monotherapy in the early stages of Parkinson's disease or in advanced stages in conjunction with levodopa. Its side effects include flu-like symptoms, joint pain, and depression. Other side effects are similar to levodopa.

- Should be stopped 2 weeks before general anesthesia.
- May interact with MAO inhibitors.

(b) Selegiline (Eldepryl®)

- Starting dose is 5 mg once daily in the morning, increased to 5 mg twice daily. Last dose should be taken in afternoon to avoid insomnia.
- May be used as monotherapy in early stage of Parkinson's disease or in advanced stages in conjunction with levodopa. Its side effects include insomnia. Other side effects are similar to levodopa.

5. *Amantadine (Symmetrel®)*

Starting dose is 100 mg three times daily. It may be used in early stage of Parkinson's disease for resting tremor and in advanced stages for dyskinesias. Its side effects include livedo reticularis, visual hallucinations, and leg edema.

6. *Anticholinergics*

(a) Trihexyphenidyl (Artane®)

- Usual dose is 1–5 mg three times daily. It is used infrequently and mainly for resting tremor in Parkinson's disease. It is also avoided in elderly patients due to increased risk of anticholinergic side effects which include dry mouth, urinary problems, confusion, and glaucoma.

(b) Benztropine (Cogentin®)

- Usual dose is 0.5–2 mg two times daily. Use and side effects are similar to trihexyphenidyl.

1.7 Rehabilitation Treatment of Parkinson's Disease

Physiotherapy, speech therapy, as well as occupational therapy have an important adjunctive role in the treatment of Parkinson's disease.

1.8   Surgical Treatments of Parkinson's Disease

Medically refractory cases of Parkinson's disease with motor fluctuations, severe levodopa-induced dyskinesia, and significant disability from their symptoms benefit from the surgical treatments. Deep brain stimulation helps mainly those symptoms which respond to dopaminergic treatment. The total dose of levodopa required by the patient can be effectively reduced. Stimulation of two targets, the subthalamic nucleus (STN) and globus pallidus pars interna (GPi) can result in improvement of most of the motor symptoms of Parkinson's disease. The optimal target for PD therapy, STN or GPI, has not been established yet.

Patients with advanced liver, renal, coronary artery disease, pulmonary conditions, severe dementia, depression, or cancer are not considered good candidates for the surgical procedures. The patients are assessed by a multidisciplinary team. Adverse effects include infection, device malfunction, seizures, depression, anxiety, apathy, hypomania, hallucination, and cognitive dysfunction.

1.9   Cerebellar Tremor

Cerebellar tremor causes a slow oscillation of approximately 3–5 Hz in a horizontal plane. Tremor of the head and trunk may be caused by midline cerebellar lesions. It is not a true tremor because in most cases it is ataxia of the affected limb or body part. It is important to distinguish this tremor from cerebellar outflow tremor. Cerebellar tremor poorly responds to surgical treatments.

1.10   Dystonic Tremor

Dystonic tremor is a postural and/or a kinetic tremor which is usually not seen during complete repose and occurs in a body part or limb affected by dystonia. These tremors are usually focal with irregular amplitudes and variable frequencies, and many patients have a null point, where tremor completely disappears. Patients with cervical dystonia may have a head tremor, and they may find that touching certain parts of their head or face with their hand or finger may help in transiently diminishing the amplitude of the tremor. This phenomenon is known as "sensory trick" and is helpful in establishing the diagnosis of dystonic head tremor.

Patients with segmental dystonia may have both head and arm tremor. Postural hand tremor may be associated with cervical dystonia in about 30 % of patients. Although this condition may become apparent at any age, symptoms usually begin between the ages of 20 and 60 years. Women are affected twice more than men. Some patients with otherwise typical ET develop focal dystonia in a segment, which is not affected by tremor. The term dystonic tremor is also used for these patients, and it remains controversial whether this is a subtype of ET.

1.11   Task-Specific Tremor

This type of tremor involves the highly skilled professional activities, and the more common daily motor activities or movements such as eating, drinking fluids, or handling other objects are not affected. Patients who usually suffer from this type of tremor are those who perform motor activities at the highest level, such as musicians or sportsmen. It is controversial whether a task-specific tremor is a variant of an essential tremor or a dystonic tremor. Task-specific writing tremor is one of the most common task-specific tremors. *Task-specific writing tremor type A* occurs only during the act of writing, while the *task-specific writing tremor type B* occurs even when the hand assumes the writing position

Primary writing tremor is characterized by its large amplitude and occurs at a frequency of 5–6 Hz. This tremor only occurs during the act of writing or when the hand assumes a writing position and only involves the affected arm. Primary writing tremor is often unilateral but may involve the other side in some advanced cases. This tremor may be difficult to distinguish from writer's dystonia or essential tremor that is aggravated by writing. This type of tremor may respond to thalamic stimulation.

1.12   Medication-Induced Tremor

Medication-induced tremors have an onset that is temporally related to the history of medication usage. The tremor is usually symmetrical, and there may be more than one type of tremor present simultaneously. Tardive tremor is seen in the context of long duration of use of antipsychotics. Dopamine antagonists and dopamine-depleting drugs, especially with prolonged use, can cause tremor and parkinsonism with an incidence ranging from 10 to 60 % depending on the type of drug used. However, in some cases the tremor and parkinsonism can even emerge within several days of treatment with these drugs. About 10% of patients may develop persistent and progressive tremors and parkinsonism despite the discontinuation of the causative drug. Females appear to have a higher incidence than males.

The following are the medications which have been implicated in the causation of drug-induced tremors and parkinsonism.

1.12.1   Frequent Causes of Drug-Induced Tremors and Parkinsonism

1. *Typical antipsychotics*
   (a) Phenothiazines: chlorpromazine, triflupromazine, thioridazine fluphenazine, piperazine, promethazine, prochlorperazine, and perphenazine
   (b) Butyrophenones: haloperidol and droperidol
   (c) Dibenzazepine: loxapine
   (d) Diphenylbutylpiperidine: pimozide
   (e) Indolines: molindone
   (f) Substituted benzamides: metoclopramide, cisapride, veralipride, alizapride, and remoxipride
   (g) Thioxanthenes: chlorprothixene and thiothixene

2. *Atypical antipsychotics*

   • Risperidone and olanzapine

3. *Dopamine-depleting drugs*

   • Tetrabenazine and reserpine

1.12.2   Infrequent Causes of Drug-Induced Tremors and Parkinsonism

(a) Antidepressants: SSRIs, e.g., paroxetine, citalopram, fluoxetine, and sertraline
(b) Immunosuppressants: cyclophosphamide, cytosine arabinoside, and cyclosporine
(c) Mood stabilizers: lithium and valproate
(d) Antihypertensives: calcium channel blockers, diltiazem, nifedipine, verapamil, amlodipine, flunarizine, and cinnarizine
(e) Other agents: amphotericin B, amiodarone, meperidine, disulfiram, and methyldopa

Lithium and valproic acid are associated with postural and kinetic tremor in many clinical settings.

1.13   Primary Orthostatic Tremor

Primary orthostatic tremor is usually a lower extremity tremor, which occurs upon standing and disappears with walking (involves the legs and trunk). This type of tremor has a very high frequency of 14–18 Hz, with bursts of motor unit activity. Upper limbs, if become involved in the tremor, are synchronous with the lower extremities. It may cause patients to feel unsteady while standing but not while walking except in severe cases. These patients do not have a problem sitting or lying down. The diagnosis of this tremor can be confirmed by electromyographic discharges of a 14–18 Hz pattern. All of the muscles in the legs, trunk, and arm show this pattern, which is absent during sitting and lying down. Presence of a coherent high-frequency electromyographic discharge pattern, in all the involved muscles, suggests that orthostatic tremor is a central tremor. This tremor can be treated with clonazepam, primidone, and gabapentin although the response may not be great.

1.14   Holmes Tremor

Holmes tremor or midbrain tremor was first described by Gordon Holmes in 1904. It is an undulating tremor, present at rest but increases in severity through sustained posture of upper extremities and is further amplified during active movement. This tremor is characterized by a frequency of 2–5 Hz but has high amplitude and is extremely debilitating. The kinetic component is greater than postural component, and the postural component is greater than the resting component. Another feature is more pronounced involvement of the proximal upper extremity segment in the generation of tremor, which is different from typical distal ET or PD tremor.

Holmes tremor is likely to be caused by interruption of fibers in the superior cerebellar peduncle which carry cerebellothalamic and cerebello-olivary projections in the midbrain contralateral to the affected limb. Terms like rubral tremor or cerebellar outflow tremor have also been used for this type of tremor. Some of the known causes of midbrain tremor include cerebrovascular accidents, multiple sclerosis, infection, hypoxia, trauma, and cystic lesions which interrupt fibers of the superior cerebellar peduncle carrying cerebellothalamic and cerebello-olivary projections in the midbrain. Ataxia and weakness may be accompanied features with Holmes tremors.

Treatment of Holmes tremor is challenging as it responds poorly to medical treatments. There is only a partial response to pharmacological agents. Some evidence of partial improvement with anticholinergic therapy, dopaminergic agents alone or in combination with isoniazid is also found in literature. However, a significant response to stereotactic thalamotomy and DBS in ventralis intermedius nucleus of contralateral thalamus may be seen. As the treatment of midbrain tremor is difficult, surgery is an option early on in this condition. Botulinum toxin injections may help in damp-ening the amplitude of the tremor but may result in weakness of the affected hand and arm muscles. The effect of botuli-num toxin usually lasts for about 3 months, and the injections have to be repeated. In this type of tremor, treatment should be assessed on a case by case basis, and all options should be considered after a risk-benefit assessment.

1.15   Alcoholic Tremor

Alcoholic tremor occurs in the lower body parts such as in the legs. It is usually 3 Hz in oscillation and can be differentiated from essential tremor by lack of family history of tremor and a greater responsiveness to propranolol.

1.16   Fragile X Tremor/Ataxia Syndrome (FTAX)

Fragile X-associated tremor/ataxia syndrome usually affects individuals above the age of 50 years. About two thirds of patients manifest a kinetic tremor. In fragile X syndrome A and fragile X-associated tremor/ataxia syndrome, there is expansion of CGG repeats of the FMR1 gene on chromosome Xq27.3 in the premutation range. The normal number of CGG repeats is 6–50, the premutation range 50–200 repeats, and fragile X syn-drome patients have 200–1,500 repeats. About 1 in 1,000 males and 1 in 250 females may carry the fragile X syndrome A pre-mutation. The fragile X-associated tremor/ataxia syndrome has a prevalence of 1 in 3,000 men above the age of 50.

It is the most common form of X-linked mental retarda-tion, and there may be a family history of mental retardation. Typical scenario involves grandsons with fragile X transmit-ted through FTAX patients' daughters, because of expansion of CGG repeats in successive generations.

FTAX patients may have an impaired gait and fine motor skills, cerebellar ataxia, fluctuating weakness, sensory symptoms, sexual dysfunction, bladder or bowel dysfunction, parkinsonism, weakness of proximal lower extremities, and cognitive dysfunction. Tremor in FTAX is mostly postural and action with occasional presence of resting tremor in advanced stages of the disease. The patients with cognitive dysfunction have impaired executive functioning with relative sparing of language and visuospatial skills. Females with the premutation may have mild cognitive dysfunction with impairment of visual attention. In addition, females may have premature ovarian failure and early menopause. Females with fragile X-associated tremor/ataxia syndrome have also been described contrary to previous reports. MRI is typical for T2 hyperintensity of the middle cerebellar peduncles, which has been suggested as a diagnostic criterion for FTAX.

1.17   Psychogenic Tremor

Psychogenic tremors have variable erratic frequency and fluctuations in amplitude. The tremor may go into remission for variable periods of time but may reoccur spontaneously. Usually the frequency is 6 Hz or less. The frequency of psychogenic tremor may correspond to the frequency of voluntary repetitive movements of the ipsilateral or contralateral limb. The patients may show an inability to perform the voluntary repetitive movements at a certain frequency requested by the examiner. However, the psychogenic tremor is a diagnosis of exclusion. If the abnormal movement is not rhythmical, the author prefers not to use the word tremor in the final diagnosis and rather describes the abnormal movement in detail. The following features may be helpful in diagnosing psychogenic tremor:

1. Abrupt onset of symptoms
2. Abnormal posture or movements disappearing with distraction
3. Inconsistent movements or postures which change characteristics over time
4. Incongruous movements and postures which do not fit with recognized physiological patterns

5. Spontaneous remissions of symptoms
6. Presence of additional abnormal movements not consistent with the basic abnormal movement pattern or not congruous with a known movement disorder such as rhythmical shaking, slowness in carrying out voluntary movement, and excessive startle in response to sudden, unexpected noise, or threatening movement
7. Presence of features of a paroxysmal disorder
8. Resolution of symptoms in response to placebo, suggestion, or psychotherapy

Bibliography

Bain PG, Findley LJ, Thompson PD, et al. A study of hereditary essential tremor. Brain. 1994;117:805–24.

Bain P, Brin M, Deuschl G, et al. Criteria for the diagnosis of essential tremor. Neurology. 2000;54:S7.

Barbanti P, Fabbrini G, Pauletti C, Defazio G, Cruccu G, Berardelli A. Headache in cranial and cervical dystonia. Neurology. 2005;64:1308–9.

Benabid AL, Pollak P, Gao D, et al. Chronic electrical stimulation of the ventralis intermedius nucleus of the thalamus as a treatment of movement disorders. J Neurosurg. 1996;84:203–14.

Benito-Leon J, Louis ED, Bermejo-Pareja F. Population-based case–control study of cognitive function in essential tremor. Neurology. 2006;66: 69–74.

Berry-Kravis E, Lewin F, Wuu J, et al. Tremor and ataxia in fragile X premutation carriers: blinded videotape study. Ann Neurol. 2003;53:616–23.

Bradley GW, Daroff R, Fenichel G, Marsden D. Neurology in clinical practice. 5th ed. Butlerworth & Heinmann. Oxford, UK; 2007

Brin MF, Koller W. Epidemiology and genetics of essential tremor. Mov Disord. 2000;13(Supplement 3):55–63.

Busenbark KL, Nash J, Nash S, Hubble JP, Koller WC. Is essential tremor benign? Neurology. 1991;41:1982–3.

Cooper C, Evidente VG, Hentz JG, Adler CH, Caviness JN, Gwinn-Hardy K. The effect of temperature on hand function in patients with tremor. J Hand Ther. 2000;13:276–88.

Deuschl G, Elble RJ. The pathophysiology of essential tremor. Neurology. 2000;54:S14–20.

Deuschl G, Heinen F, Guschlbauer B, Schneider S, Glocker FX, Lucking CH. Hand tremor in patients with spasmodic torticollis. Mov Disord. 1997;12:547–52.

Deuschl G, Koster B, Lucking CH, Scheidt C. Diagnostic and pathophysiological aspects of psychogenic tremors. Mov Disord. 1998;13:294–302.

Elble RJ. The role of aging in the clinical expression of essential tremor. Exp Gerontol. 1995;30:337–47.

Elble RJ. Tremor in ostensibly normal elderly people. Mov Disord. 1998;13:457–64.

Elble RJ. Essential tremor frequency decreases with time. Neurology. 2000;55:1547–51.

Elble RJ. Essential tremor is a monosymptomatic disorder. Mov Disord. 2002;17:633–7.

Elble RJ. Characteristics of physiologic tremor in young and elderly adults. Clin Neurophysiol. 2003;114:624–35.

Elble RJ. Report from a U.S. conference on essential tremor. Mov Disord. 2006;21:2052–61.

Gasparini M, Bonifati V, Fabrizio E, et al. Frontal lobe dysfunction in essential tremor: a preliminary study. J Neurol. 2001;248:399–402.

Gironell A, Kulisevsky J, Pascual-Sedano B, Barbanoj M. Routine neurophysiologic tremor analysis as a diagnostic tool for essential tremor: a prospective study. J Clin Neurophysiol. 2004;21:446–50.

Goetz CG, Pappert EJ. Textbook of clinical neurology. 2nd ed. Philadelphia: Saunders; 1999.

Gulcher JR, Jonsson P, Kong A, et al. Mapping of a familial essential tremor gene, FET1, to chromosome 3q13. Nat Genet. 1997;17:84–7.

Hagerman RJ, Leavitt BR, Farzin F, et al. Fragile-X-associated tremor/ataxia syndrome (FXTAS) in females with the FMR1 premutation. Am J Hum Genet. 2004;74:1051–6.

Hall DA, Berry-Kravis E, Jacquemont S, et al. Initial diagnoses given to persons with the fragile X associated tremor/ataxia syndrome (FXTAS). Neurology. 2005;65:299–301.

Hardesty DE, Maraganore DM, Matsumoto JY, Louis ED. Increased risk of head tremor in women with essential tremor: longitudinal data from the Rochester Epidemiology Project. Mov Disord. 2004;19:529–33.

Hellwig B, Häussler S, Schelter B, et al. Tremor-correlated cortical activity in essential tremor. Lancet. 2001;357:519–23.

Helmchen C, Hagenow A, Miesner J, et al. Eye movement abnormalities in essential tremor may indicate cerebellar dysfunction. Brain. 2003;126:1319–32.

Higgins JJ, Pho LT, Nee LE. A gene (ETM) for essential tremor maps to chromosome 2p22-p25. Mov Disord. 1997;6:859–64.

Higgins JJ, Lombardi RQ, Pucilowska J, Jankovic J, Tan EK, Rooney JP. A variant in the HS1-BP3 gene is associated with familial essential tremor. Neurology. 2005;64:417–21.

Higgins JJ, Lombardi RQ, Pucilowska J, Jankovic J, Golbe LI, Verhagen L. HS1-BP3 gene variant is common in familial essential tremor. Mov Disord. 2006;21:306–9.

Hsu YD, Chang MK, Sung SC, Hsein HH, Deng JC. Essential tremor: clinical, electromyographical and pharmacological studies in 146 Chinese patients. Chung Hua I Hsueh Tsa Chih (Taipei). 1990;45:93–9.

Hua SE, Lenz FA. Posture-related oscillations in human cerebellar thalamus in essential tremor are enabled by voluntary motor circuits. J Neurophysiol. 2005;93:117–27.

Jacquemont S, Hagerman RJ, Leehey M, et al. Fragile X premutation tremor/ataxia syndrome: molecular, clinical, and neuroimaging correlates. Am J Hum Genet. 2003;72:869–78.

Jain S, Lo SE, Louis ED. Common misdiagnosis of a common neurological disorder: how are we misdiagnosing essential tremor? Arch Neurol. 2006;63:1100–4.

Jankovic J. Essential tremor: a heterogenous disorder. Mov Disord. 2002;17:638–44.

Jankovic J. Botulinum toxin in clinical practice. J Neurol Neurosurg Psychiatry. 2004;75:951–7.

Jankovic J, Tolosa E. Parkinson's disease and movement disorder. 5th ed. Philadelphia: Lippincott Williams and Wilkins; 2007.

Khan W, Rana AQ. Dopamine agonist induced compulsive eating behaviour in a Parkinson's disease patient. Pharm World Sci. 2010;32:114–6.

Khan W, Naz S, Rana AQ. Shortness of breath, a 'wearing-off' symptom in Parkinson's disease. Clin Drug Investig. 2009;29:689–91.

Kim YJ, Pakiam AS, Lang AE. Historical and clinical features of psychogenic tremor: a review of 70 cases. Can J Neurol Sci. 1999;26:190–5.

Klebe S, Stolze H, Grensing K, Volkmann J, Wenzelburger R, Deuschl G. Influence of alcohol on gait in patients with essential tremor. Neurology. 2005;65:96–101.

Koster B, Lauk M, Timmer J, et al. Involvement of cranial muscles and high intermuscular coherence in orthostatic tremor. Ann Neurol. 1999;45:384–8.

Koster B, Deuschl G, Lauk M, Timmer J, Guschlbauer B, Lücking CH. Essential tremor and cerebellar dysfunction: abnormal ballistic movements. J Neurol Neurosurg Psychiatry. 2002;73:400–5.

Kovach MJ, Ruiz J, Kimonis K, et al. Genetic heterogeneity in autosomal dominant essential tremor. Genet Med. 2001;3:197–9.

Kumar R, Lozano AM, Sime E, Lang AE. Long-term follow-up of thalamic deep brain stimulation for essential and parkinsonian tremor. Neurology. 2003;61:1601–4.

Leehey MA, Hagerman RJ, Landau WM, et al. Tremor/ataxia syndrome in fragile X carrier males. Mov Disord. 2002;17:744–5.

Lombardi WJ, Woolston DJ, Roberts JW, Gross RE. Cognitive deficits in patients with essential tremor. Neurology. 2001;57:785–90.

Lorenz D, Frederiksen H, Moises H, Kopper F, Deuschl G, Christensen K. High concordance for essential tremor in monozygotic twins of old age. Neurology. 2004;62:208–11.

Louis ED. Etiology of essential tremor: should we be searching for environmental causes? Mov Disord. 2001;16:822–9.

Louis ED, Ottman R. Study of possible factors associated with age of onset in essential tremor. Mov Disord. 2006;21:1980–6.

Louis ED, Ford B, Lee H, Andrews H, Camero G. Diagnostic criteria for essential tremor: a population perspective. Arch Neurol. 1998a;55:823–8.

Louis ED, Ford B, Pullman S, Baron K. How normal is 'normal'? Mild tremor in a multiethnic cohort of normal subjects. Arch Neurol. 1998b;55:222–7.

Louis ED, Ottman R, Hauser WA. How common is the most common adult movement disorder? Estimates of the prevalence of essential tremor throughout the world. Mov Disord. 1998c;13:5–10.

Louis ED, Wendt KJ, Pullman SL, Ford B. Is essential tremor symmetric? Observational data from a community- based study of essential tremor. Arch Neurol. 1998d;55:1553–9.

Louis ED, Ford B, Barnes LF. Clinical subtypes of essential tremor. Arch Neurol. 2000a;57:1194–8.

Louis ED, Wendt KJ, Ford B. Senile tremor: what is the prevalence and severity of tremor in older adults? Gerontology. 2000b;46:12–6.

Louis ED, Dure LS, Pullman S. Essential tremor in childhood: a series of nineteen cases. Mov Disord. 2001a;16:921–3.

Louis ED, Ford B, Frucht S, Barnes LF, Tang MX, Ottman R. Risk of tremor and impairment from tremor in relatives of patients with essential tremor: a community-based family study. Ann Neurol. 2001b;49:761–9.

Louis ED, Fernandez-Alvarez E, Dure 4th LS, Frucht S, Ford B. Association between male gender and pediatric essential tremor. Mov Disord. 2005;20:904–6.

Louis ED, Rios E, Applegate LM, Hernandez NC, Andrews HF. Jaw tremor: prevalence and clinical correlates in three essential tremor case samples. Mov Disord. 2006a;21:1872–8.

Louis ED, Vonsattel JP, Honig LS, et al. Essential tremor associated with pathologic changes in the cerebellum. Arch Neurol. 2006b;63:1189–93.

Louis ED, Vonsattel JP, Honig LS, et al. Neuropathologic findings in essential tremor. Neurology. 2006c;66:1756–9.

Ma S, Davis TL, Blair MA, et al. Familial essential tremor with apparent autosomal dominant inheritance: should we also consider other inheritance modes? Mov Disord. 2006;21:1368–74.

Murata J, Kitagawa M, Uesugi H, et al. Electrical stimulation of the posterior subthalamic area for the treatment of intractable proximal tremor. J Neurosurg. 2003;99:708–15.

O'Suilleabhain PE, Matsumoto JY. Time-frequency analysis of tremors. Brain. 1998;121:2127–34.

Obwegeser AA, Uitti RJ, Turk MF, Strongosky AJ, Wharen RE. Thalamic stimulation for the treatment of midline tremors in essential tremor patients. Neurology. 2000;54:2342–4.

Ohye C, Shibazaki T, Zhang J, Andou Y. Thalamic lesions produced by gamma thalamotomy for movement disorders. J Neurosurg. 2002;97 (5 Suppl):600–6.

Ondo WG, Jankovic J, Connor GS, et al. Topiramate in essential tremor: a double-blind, placebo-controlled trial. Neurology. 2006;66:672–7.

Pahapill PA, Levy R, Dostrovsky JO, et al. Tremor arrest with thalamic microinjections of muscimol in patients with essential tremor. Ann Neurol. 1999;46:249–52.

Papavassiliou E, Rau G, Heath S, et al. Thalamic deep brain stimulation for essential tremor: relation of lead location to outcome. Neurosurgery. 2004;54:1120–30.

Paulson GW. Benign essential tremor in childhood: symptoms, pathogenesis, treatment. Clin Pediatr (Phila). 1976;15:67–70.

Pellecchia MT, Varrone A, Annesi G, et al. Parkinsonism and essential tremor in a family with pseudo-dominant inheritance of PARK2: an FP-CIT SPECT study. Mov Disord. 2006;22:559–63.

Phibbs FT, Fang JY, Cooper MK, et al. Prevalence of unilateral tremor in autosomal dominant essential tremor. Mov Disord. 2009;24: 108–11.

Plaha P, Patel NK, Gill SS. Stimulation of the subthalamic region for essential tremor. J Neurosurg. 2004;101:48–54.

Raethjen J, Kopper F, Govindan RB, Volkmann J, Deuschl G. Two different pathogenetic mechanisms in psychogenic tremor. Neurology. 2004; 63:812–5.

Rajput A, Robinson CA, Rajput AH. Essential tremor course and disability: a clinicopathologic study of 20 cases. Neurology. 2004;62:932–6.

Rana AQ. An introduction to essential tremor. Bloomington: iUniverse Publishing; 2010.

Ray LW, Koller WC. Movement disorders, neurologic principles and practice. 2nd ed. New York: McGraw-Hill; 1997.

Rolands LP, editor. Merritt's textbook of neurology. 10th ed. New York: Lippincott Williams & Wilkins; 2000.

Sahin HA, Terzi M, Ucak S, Yapici O, Basoglu T, Onar M. Frontal functions in young patients with essential tremor: a case comparison study. J Neuropsychiatry Clin Neurosci. 2006;18:64–72.

Samii A, Pal PK, Schulzer M, Mak E, Tsui JK. Post-traumatic cervical dystonia: a distinct entity? Can J Neurol Sci. 2000;27:55–9.

Sander HW, Masdeu JC, Tavoulareas G, Walters A, Zimmerman T, Chokroverty S. Orthostatic tremor: an electrophysiological analysis. Mov Disord. 1998;13:735–8.

Schols L, Bauer P, Schmidt T, Schulte T, Riess O. Autosomal dominant cerebellar ataxias: clinical features, genetics, and pathogenesis. Lancet Neurol. 2004;3:291–304.

Schrag A, Munchau A, Bhatia KP, Quinn NP, Marsden CD. Essential tremor: an overdiagnosed condition? J Neurol. 2000;247:955–9.

Schuurman PR, Bosch DA, Bossuyt PM, et al. A comparison of continuous thalamic stimulation and thalamotomy for suppression of severe tremor. N Engl J Med. 2000;342:461–8.

Shah M, Findley L, Muhammed N, Hawkes C. Olfaction is normal in essential tremor and can be used to distinguish it from Parkinson's disease. Mov Disord. 2005;20 Suppl 10:S166.

Shatunov A, Jankovic J, Elble R, et al. A variant in the HS1-BP3 gene is associated with familial essential tremor. Neurology. 2005;65(12):1995.

Siderowf A, Gollump SM, Stern MB, Baltuch GH, Riina HA. Emergence of complex, involuntary movements after gamma knife radiosurgery for essential tremor. Mov Disord. 2001;16:965–7.

Singh NN, Thomas FP. Fragile X-associated tremor/ataxia syndrome. In: Greenamyre JT, editor-in-chief. MedLink Neurology. San Diego: MedLink Corporation; 2008. Available at www.medlink.com.

Soland VL, Bhatia KP, Volonte MA, Marsden CD. Focal task-specific tremors. Mov Disord. 1996;11:665–70.

Stemp LI, Taswell C. Spastic torticollis during general anesthesia: case report and review of receptor mechanisms. Anesthesiology. 1991;75:365–6.

Stolze H, Petersen G, Raethjen J, Wenzelburger R, Deuschl G. The gait disorder of advanced essential tremor. Brain. 2001;124:2278–86.

Stover NP, Okun MS, Evatt ML, Raju DV, Bakay RA, Vitek JL. Stimulation of the subthalamic nucleus in a patient with Parkinson disease and essential tremor. Arch Neurol. 2005;62:141–3.

Sydow O, Thobois S, Alesch F, Speelman JD. Multicentre European study of thalamic stimulation in essential tremor: a six year follow up. J Neurol Neurosurg Psychiatry. 2003;74:1387–91.

Taha JM, Janszen MA, Favre J. Thalamic deep brain stimulation for the treatment of head, voice, and bilateral limb tremor. J Neurosurg. 1999; 91:68–72.

Tan EK, Zhao Y, Puong KY, et al. Fragile X premutation alleles in SCA, ET, and parkinsonism in an Asian cohort. Neurology. 2004;63:362–3.

Tan EK, Lum SY, Prakash KM. Clinical features of childhood onset essential tremor. Eur J Neurol. 2006;13:1302–5.

Tanner CM, Goldman SM, Lyons KE, et al. Essential tremor in twins: an assessment of genetic versus environmental determinants of etiology. Neurology. 2001;57:1389–91.

Ushe M, Mink JW, Revilla FJ, et al. Effect of stimulation frequency on tremor suppression in essential tremor. Mov Disord. 2004;19:1163–8.

Zackowski KM, Bastian AJ, Hakimian S, et al. Thalamic stimulation reduces essential tremor but not the delayed antagonist muscle timing. Neurology. 2002;58:402–10.

Zesiewicz TA, Elble R, Louis ED, et al. Practice parameter: therapies for essential tremor: report of the Quality Standards Subcommittee of the American Academy of Neurology. Neurology. 2005;64:2008–20.

Chapter 2
Dystonia

Abstract Dystonia is an involuntary movement characterized by sustained, patterned, and repetitive muscle contractions of opposing muscles, causing abnormal postures
and hyperkinetic jerky movements of affected body parts.
This chapter reviews main characteristics of dystonia,
classification of dystonias based on spread of symptoms
(focal, segmental, hemidystonia, generalized dystonia) and
etiology (genetic and acquired dystonias). We discuss main
clinical features of the most common types of dystonias,
their differential diagnosis, and main therapeutic options,
including therapy with botulinum toxins and deep brain
stimulation. Additional emphasis is on treatable causes
of dystonia, such as levodopa-responsive dystonia and
Wilson's disease.

Keywords Dystonia • Therapy • Botulinum toxin • Deep
brain stimulation

Dystonia is defined as involuntary, sustained, patterned, and
repetitive muscle contractions of opposing muscles, resulting
in twisting or spasmodic movements, or abnormal postures of
the involved body parts.

A.Q. Rana, P. Hedera, *Differential Diagnosis of Movement*   43
Disorders in Clinical Practice, DOI 10.1007/978-3-319-01607-8_2,
© Springer International Publishing Switzerland 2014

2.1   Classification

Dystonia can be classified into the following types:

(A) *According to body distribution*

1. Focal dystonia

   - Involves one single body part (e.g., task-specific dystonia, such as writer's dystonia)

2. Segmental dystonia

   - Involves one or more contiguous body parts (e.g., craniocervical dystonia such as Meige syndrome)

3. Multifocal dystonia

   - Involves two or more noncontiguous body parts

4. Hemidystonia

   - Involves one side of body and is usually related to structural lesion in basal ganglia

5. Generalized dystonia

   - Involves whole body diffusely

(B) *According to the age of onset*

1. Infantile (0–12 years)
2. Juvenile (12–20 years)
3. Adult (>20 years)

   Childhood-onset dystonia frequently becomes generalized, whereas adult-onset dystonia is more likely to remain focal or segmental.

(C) *According to etiology*

1. Primary childhood onset such as DYT1 and adult onset, such as adult-onset idiopathic focal cervical dystonia
2. Secondary or acquired, such as drug induced

3. Dystonia-plus conditions such as dystonia-parkinsonism and dystonia-myoclonus
4. Inherited, such as classic Oppenheim's dystonia DYT1
5. Psychogenic
6. Pseudodystonia
7. Others such as musician's dystonia, writer's dystonia, blepharospasm, spasmodic dysphonia, and cervical dystonia

(D) *According to the duration of symptoms*

1. Continual, which can be primary or secondary

   (a) Primary

      (i)   Focal such as blepharospasm, writer's dystonia, cervical dystonia, foot dystonia, oromandibular dystonia
      (ii) Segmental such as cranial or brachial dystonia
      (iii) Centralized such as torsion dystonia

   (b) Secondary

      (i) Unilateral such as hemidystonia seen in stroke, trauma, and tumors
      (ii) Focal, segmental, multifocal, or generalized

2. Fluctuating

   (i) Diurnal and paroxysmal, such as kinesigenic and non-kinesigenic

2.1.1   Special Features of Dystonia

1. Motor trick (e.g., jaw movement relieves blepharospasm)
2. Sensory trick (e.g., touching the side of face with one finger brings the head in neutral position)
3. Pain (e.g., neck pain in cervical dystonia)
4. Tremor (e.g., head tremor in cervical dystonia)

2.2   Investigations

In many cases where the diagnosis is apparent, investigations are not required. The following investigations may be considered in atypical cases:

1. MRI or CT scan of the head.
2. MRI or CT scan of the craniocervical junction.
3. EMG studies in difficult cases for muscle localization for botulinum toxin treatment.
4. If patient is young and Wilson's disease is suspected, consider screening by the serum ceruloplasmin, 24 h urine copper, and slit lamp examination for Kayser-Fleischer rings.

Although the diagnosis of dystonia is made clinically, there are no confirmatory laboratory tests or imaging available. A detailed drug history should be taken in order to exclude drug-induced dystonia. In patients with onset before the age of 40, Wilson's disease should be ruled out. Before making a diagnosis of dystonia, secondary causes of dystonia such as the following should be excluded:

1. History of possible etiologic factor (e.g., head and neck trauma, peripheral trauma, encephalitis, toxin exposure, or drug exposure)
2. Presence of other neurological condition (e.g., dementia, seizures, ataxia, weakness, spasticity)
3. Hemidystonia due to central lesion
4. Onset of rest, instead of action, dystonia
5. Abnormal brain imaging such as MRI

During the physical examination, the examiner checks range of different movements of the affected body region, palpates the muscles of head and neck region which may be involved, and may need to prepare video recordings for comparison at future visits. Author finds it helpful to have the patient close his/her eyes and let the head to assume the most comfortable position without any active movement or resistance.

2.3 Causes

The common types of childhood-onset and adult-onset dystonias are discussed below, although there may be some overlap between these two classifications.

2.3.1 Primary Idiopathic Torsion Dystonia (DYT-1)

Primary idiopathic torsion dystonia is an autosomal dominant disorder. Although primary idiopathic torsion dystonia may affect various ethnic groups, it is most prevalent in the Ashkenazi Jews, affecting 1 in 6,000 individuals. The mean age at onset is 12.5 ± 8.2 years. The onset, however, is rare after the age of 29. In primary idiopathic torsion dystonia, the DYTI gene mutation on chromosome 9q has been known. The penetrance rate is around 30–40 %, and the only abnormality is a deletion of one of a pair of GAG triplets in the ATP-binding protein, torsin A.

The symptoms of primary idiopathic torsion dystonia begin in a leg or arm and spread to the larynx or neck. When primary idiopathic torsion dystonia starts in a leg, it may progress to generalized dystonia in majority of cases. However, when it starts in an arm, it may progress to generalized dystonia in about half of the cases. With leg involvement, action dystonia results in an abnormal twisting of the leg when the patient walks forward, even though running, walking backward, or dancing may still be normal. Patients may find it difficult to place the heel on the ground, due to the affected distal muscles. As primary idiopathic torsion dystonia progresses, the movements may appear when the leg is at rest; the foot is usually plantar flexed and turned inwards.

With arm involvement, primary idiopathic torsion dystonia can interfere with writing and other activities. With progression, the dystonia may be present even when the arm is at rest, and the dystonia may spread to the other arm or occasionally to the neighboring body parts.

With time the primary idiopathic torsion dystonia may spread to other parts of the body, proceeding from focal to segmental to generalized dystonia. The trunk may develop abnormal posture, with speech problems and facial grimacing, albeit infrequently. Although muscle power and tone may be normal, the involuntary movements interfere with daily activities. The rate of progression of dystonia is variable and may be most severe within the first 5–10 years. Spasms may cause a marked distortion of the body.

2.3.2 Primary Idiopathic Dystonia (DYT-6)

This is the second most common form of dystonia, caused by mutations in the *THAP1* gene on chromosome 8p. It can cause generalized, segmental, and focal dystonia. It was first reported in families with the onset in the second decade and the onset of dystonia in the extremities, similar to DYT-1. However, subsequent genetic analysis identified patients with craniocervical onset, including isolated focal dystonia, laryngeal dystonia, or blepharospasm; their age of onset varied from the second to sixth decades.

2.3.3 Dopa-Responsive Dystonia

Around 10 % of patients with childhood-onset dystonia may have dopa-responsive dystonia or *Segawa disease*. Dopa-responsive dystonia may manifest between ages 6 and 16, although symptoms may occur at any age. Dopa-responsive dystonia affects girls four times more than boys and is not known to have a higher occurrence in any specific ethnic groups. Dopa-responsive dystonia is different from other childhood dystonias due to the presence of cogwheel rigidity, bradykinesia, impaired postural reflexes, and hyperreflexia, mainly in the legs. Patients have diurnal fluctuations with improvement of symptoms after sleep and deterioration as the day goes on.

Distinguishing dopa-responsive dystonia from primary idiopathic torsion dystonia is important due to its good response to levodopa. Patients respond to low doses of levodopa. In childhood it may resemble cerebral palsy, and with onset in adults, it resembles parkinsonism. The main causes of dopa-responsive dystonia are various mutations of the gene for GTP cyclohydrolase I (GCHI), located at chromosome 14q22.1, and genetic label dopa-responsive dystonia is DYT5. This trait is transmitted in an autosomal dominant fashion. There is no loss of neurons within the substantia nigra pars compacta, but the cells may be immature with little neuromelanin. There is significant reduction of dopamine in the striatum in dopa-responsive dystonia; hence, it is a neurochemical rather than a neurodegenerative disease.

Atypical cases of dopa-responsive dystonia may be inherited in an autosomal recessive pattern with mutations in the gene for tyrosine hydroxylase, and the dystonia-parkinsonism starts in infancy or early childhood in these cases.

The differential diagnosis of dopa-responsive dystonia includes juvenile parkinsonism. Fluorodopa positron emission tomography is normal dopa-responsive dystonia, whereas in juvenile parkinsonism, reduction of fluorodopa uptake in the striatum may be seen. The starting dose of levodopa/carbidopa for dopa-responsive dystonia is 12.5/50 mg two or three times a day. Patients can be maintained on a dosage of 25/100 mg two or three times daily, and in contrast to PD, their levodopa dose is stable throughout the lifelong treatment.

2.3.4 Writer's Dystonia

Writer's dystonia is an adult-onset focal task-specific dystonia which affects only writing. It typically remains limited to one limb and is seen generally on the dominant side. Infrequently it may develop in the other arm as well. Treatment modalities are limited. Non-pharmacological strategies such as different writing devices and thick pens may provide some help. Botulinum toxin may offer some help in the treatment of writer's dystonia.

2.3.5   Musician's Dystonia

Musician's dystonia is seen in piano players and is also a type of adult-onset focal dystonia. Other fine motor movements with the affected hand remain normal. This may significantly interfere with the performance of these professionals. Chemodenervation with botulinum toxin may provide some relief in these patients.

2.3.6   Spasmodic Dystonia

Spasmodic dysphonia, e.g., dystonia of the vocal cords, occurs in two varieties. The more common type is called *spasmodic dysphonia*, in which the vocal cords adduct causing the voice to be strangled, coarse, and restricted with pauses. Spasmodic dysphonia may be associated with tremor of the vocal cords, and botulinum toxin can be noticeably effective in treating spasmodic dysphonia. DYT-6 can present as an isolated spasmodic dysphonia.

2.3.7   Blepharospasm

Blepharospasm is a focal dystonia which occurs more frequently in women than in men. The onset is generally after the age of 50 years. Initially, patients may only experience an increase in blinking. Later, patients may develop intermittent brief closure of the eyelids, which may progress to more extended and firm closure of the eyelids. Eyelid closure, however, can also be forceful and sporadic in nature. Blepharospasm can be aggravated by bright light leading to functional blindness.

A common sensory trick for temporarily relieving the symptoms is placing a finger lateral to the orbit. Although orbicularis oculi are the main muscles involved in blepharospasm, however corrugators and procerus may also be involved in many cases. Blepharospasm may cause the contraction of lower facial muscles and may become segmental by involving other cranial regions, such as the cervical muscles, tongue, jaw, or vocal cords. The grouping of blepharospasm with some other cranial dystonia is termed *Meige syndrome.*

The differential diagnosis of blepharospasm includes hemifacial spasm, which is typically unilateral in nature. Rarely is hemifacial spasm bilateral. Blinking tics can resemble blepharospasm; however, tics usually begin in childhood and can be suppressed. Botulinum toxin is the first-line treatment for blepharospasm.

2.3.8 Cervical Dystonia

Cervical dystonia is the most common form of focal dystonias. The prevalence of cervical dystonia is estimated to be between 8 and 9 cases per 100,000, and the incidence is 1.2 per 100,000. The peak age of onset of cervical dystonia is between 40 and 49 years. Females may be affected twice more than males.

Cervical dystonia is characterized by abnormally sustained muscle contractions of the head and neck region causing twisting and repetitive movements of the head and neck. The following are some of the abnormal postures of the head and neck as noted in patients with cervical dystonia:

1. Sideways or lateral turn of the head
2. Sideways or lateral tilt of head (laterocollis)
   The lateral turn and tilt of the head are the two of the most common abnormal postures observed in cervical dystonia.
3. Extension of head (retrocollis)
4. Flexion of head (anterocollis)
5. Sideways shift of head (lateral shift)
6. Anterior or posterior shift of head (sagittal shift)

In cervical dystonia, one shoulder may be more elevated and anteriorly displaced than the other one. Usually, each patient has a combination of more than one abnormal position and more than one muscle involved. Cervical dystonia may be part of certain generalized dystonias that are manifested with dystonic posturing of the body parts.

Pathophysiology

The cause of cervical dystonia remains unknown. However, it is believed that cervical dystonia is caused due to an abnormality in the basal ganglia or brainstem which results in thalamo-frontal disinhibition due to defective inhibitory control mediated by the basal ganglia.

Secondary cervical dystonia may be caused by the dopamine receptor-blocking drugs, which can also cause an acute transient dystonic reaction.

Although the majority of cases are sporadic, family history of cervical dystonia may be present in some patients. In about 10 % of patients with cervical dystonia, more than one family member is affected. Several families with adult-onset focal dystonia have been noticed to have an autosomal dominant pattern of inheritance.

A mutation of DYT7 gene locus on chromosome 18p has been suggested to be responsible for causing cervical dystonia in several large families, but in the majority of cases, there is no family history or definite inheritance pattern. DYT6 (THAP1) can also present with isolated cervical dystonia. The exact pathophysiology of cervical dystonia remains unknown.

Commonly Involved Muscle Groups

Several muscles of the head and neck region are involved in abnormal head and neck position in cervical dystonia, and each muscle has more than one action. The common neck muscles involved are sternocleidomastoid, levator scapulae, splenius capitis, trapezius, scalene, and semispinalis capitis (Figs. 2.1 and 2.2). The abnormal contractions of different combinations of these muscles cause the head to be turned or tilted to one side.

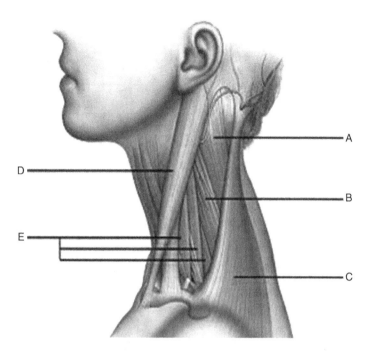

FIGURE 2.1 Muscles involved in cervical dystonia (lateral view): (A) splenius capitis muscle, (B) levator scapulae muscle, (C) trapezius muscle, (D) sternocleidomastoid muscle, and (E) scaleni muscles

Table 2.1 summarizes the anatomy and actions of the muscles commonly involved in cervical dystonia.

Symptoms of idiopathic cervical dystonia usually begin between the ages of 20 and 60 years. Initially, the disorder may start with the patient feeling the sensation of the head being pulled to one side or the other. As the time progresses, the patient may experience mild head tremor which may advance with time. In cervical dystonia, one shoulder may be elevated and displaced forward on the side towards which the chin turns.

Patients may find that touching certain parts of their head or face may help in bringing their head back into neutral position transiently. This phenomenon is known as "sensory

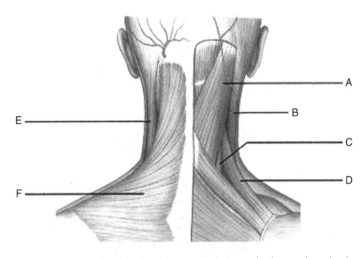

FIGURE 2.2 Muscles involved in cervical dystonia (posterior view): (A) splenius capitis muscle, (B) longissimus muscle, (C) splenius cervicis muscle, (D) levator scapulae muscle, (E) sternocleidomastoid muscle, and (F) trapezius muscle

TABLE 2.1 Muscles involved in cervical dystonia

Muscle	Anatomy	Action
Sternocleidomastoid	It has two heads; the sternal head originates from anterior and superior manubrium of the sternum. Clavicular head originates from the superior medial third of clavicle. Inserts at the lateral aspect of mastoid process and anterior half of superior nuchal line	1. Turns the head to the opposite side 2. Bend the head forward when acting together 3. Tilts the head to the ipsilateral side
Splenius capitis	Originates from the lower ligament nuchae, spinous processes, and supraspinous ligaments T1–3. Inserts at the lateral occiput between superior and inferior nuchal lines	1. Tilts the head to the ipsilateral side 2. Ipsilateral rotation of head

TABLE 2.1 (continued)

Muscle	Anatomy	Action
Semispinalis capitis	Originates from the transversal process of the lower cervical and higher thoracal column. Inserts between the superior and inferior nuchal lines	Extends the head
Scalenus anterior	Originates from the anterior tubercles of the transverse processes of the C3–6. Inserts at the scalene tubercle of the first rib	Rotates the neck to the opposite side Tilts the neck laterally and forward
Scalenus posterior	Originates from C4–6. Inserts at the second rib	Tilts the neck to the ipsilateral side
Scalenus medius	Originates from the costotransverse lamellae of the transverse processes of C2–6. Inserts at the first rib	Rotates the neck to the opposite side
Levator scapulae	Originates from the posterior tubercles of transverse processes of C1–4 and inserts at the upper part of medial border of the scapula	Elevates the ipsilateral shoulder

trick" and is helpful in establishing the diagnosis of idiopathic cervical dystonia (Fig. 2.3). Cervical dystonia is the most common focal dystonia that responds to a "sensory trick" or *geste antagoniste*. Leaning the head back against a chair or placing a hand on the top of the head may also help to relieve the symptoms. Although this observation indicates that cervical dystonia can be influenced by changing the proprioceptive input, the exact mechanism of sensory tricks is not yet known.

More than two thirds of the patients have neck pain, which may be the presenting symptom in some cases. Patients with cervical dystonia may have head tremor which could be in a

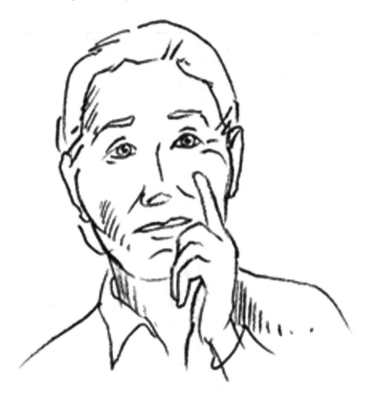

FIGURE 2.3 Touching side of face with finger helped to bring head in almost neutral position (sensory trick)

horizontal plane called a "no-no" head tremor or in a vertical plane, i.e., "yes-yes" head tremor. Postural hand tremor may be associated with cervical dystonia in about one third of patients.

In some patients the symptoms of cervical dystonia may go away for short periods of time without any treatment but may come back later. If remission occurs, it is mostly noted during the first 3 years of onset of symptoms and is more likely to occur in patients with jerky or spasmodic dystonia, as opposed to patients with a constant neck deviation. Focal cervical dystonia progresses to segmental or generalized dystonia, although rarely.

Muscle hypertrophy is a common sign of cervical dystonia and may be seen in most cases of cervical dystonia. Over two thirds of patients, particularly those with sustained head deviation, have associated neck pain. More than one third of these patients also experience head tremor, tremor of hands, or both. Approximately 20 % of patients with cervical dystonia may have blepharospasm and dystonia in muscle groups of upper limb. Swallowing may be affected in patients with extreme retrocollis. Some patients may just have the sustained turning of their head to one side, whereas other patients may have a dystonic tremor. Symptoms of cervical often worsen in stress and improve with rest and disappear in sleep.

Some patients may present with similar symptoms after trauma. These individuals have fixed torticollis with an increased tendency for laterocollis and may not respond well to treatment. The relation of cervical dystonia with trauma remains unclear. Patients with posttraumatic painful torticollis differ from typical idiopathic cervical dystonia in that usually no improvement appears during or after sleep, and there is no response to the sensory tricks.

Patients with cervical dystonia do not have any muscle contractures, but in patients with a prolonged history of cervical dystonia fixed deformities of the neck may develop overtime.

Patients with cervical dystonia have an increased risk of secondary degenerative changes of the upper cervical spine, especially on the side ipsilateral to the head tilt. This condition can contribute to the pain, poor response to botulinum toxin and surgical therapy, and limitation of head movement.

Diagnosis

Although the diagnosis of cervical dystonia is made clinically, there are no confirmatory laboratory tests or imaging available for cervical dystonia. A detailed drug history should be taken in order to exclude drug-induced dystonia. In patients with onset before the age of 40 years, Wilson's disease if suspected should be ruled out. Before making a diagnosis of cervical dystonia in a patient, secondary causes of torticollis should be excluded.

Congenital, inflammatory, or traumatic bony abnormalities in the cervical spine may be detected by X-ray or CT scan of cervical spine. Osteomyelitis, septic arthritis of the C1–C2 lateral face joint, cervical epidural abscess, and pharyngeal abscess may cause symptoms similar to torticollis. X-rays also help to assess the severity of coexisting cervical spondylosis.

CT scans and magnetic resonance imaging (MRI) usually do not provide any information regarding the diagnosis of cervical dystonia, and usually no relevant pathology is found. A variety of tumors such as cerebellar cavernous angioma, frontal meningioma, other posterior fossa tumors, spinal astrocytoma, or ependymoma may also present with symptoms similar to torticollis.

The following steps are taken for the assessment of cervical dystonia:

1. A detailed history of exposure to dopamine receptor-blocking medication and toxins. History of peripheral, head, neck, or back trauma
2. Family history of similar conditions or other movement disorders
3. Physical examination to exclude the presence of other abnormalities (e.g., impaired coordination of voluntary movements, optic atrophy, retinal abnormalities), parkinsonism, myoclonus, spasticity, focal weakness, dementia, or seizures which may suggest secondary dystonia, dystonia-plus syndromes, or heredodegenerative disorders

In children the conditions such as Sandifer syndrome may have similar presentation with tilting of the head which may relieve pain associated with hiatus hernia. In infants with torticollis, congenital shortening and fibrosis of the sternocleidomastoid muscle may be present.

Patients with cranial nerve IV palsy may have head *tilted* to the contralateral side, and the patients with cranial nerve VI may have head *turned* to the contralateral side in order to avoid diplopia. Patients with vestibular diseases may adjust their head in order to find the most comfortable position of head to avoid dizziness. Assessments by a speech-language pathologist, physical or occupational therapists, or genetic counselors may be required in some cases.

Staging of Cervical Dystonia

Due to the variations of abnormal movements caused by muscle contractions, it may be difficult to accurately measure changes in head position in patients with cervical dystonia. Nevertheless, such measurements are vital in order to assess a patient's response to various treatments.

Cervical dystonia can be measured in two ways: subjectively or objectively. Subjective measures rate a patient's pain or disability (i.e., difficulties in performing daily activities, handicaps, and social restrictions resulting from the impairments). Objective measures rate an external evaluable impairments caused by the condition. An appropriate assessment of cervical dystonia would ideally include both subjective and objective rating scales. Toronto Western Spasmodic Torticollis Rating Scale (TWSTRS) may be used in detailed assessment.

Treatment of Cervical Dystonia

The treatment of cervical dystonia may not be required if the symptoms are very mild and not bothering the patient. Once the patient has neck pain or the symptoms start interfering with activities of daily living, the treatment is initiated.

The goals of treatment for cervical dystonia are to improve the abnormal neck position and related pain, as well as preventing secondary complications such as secondary degenerative changes of cervical spine, radiculopathy, development of contractures, and cervical myelopathy.

Treatment of cervical dystonia includes chemodenervations with botulinum toxin, oral medications, and surgical treatments. Deep brain stimulation with targeting of globus pallidus pars interna is a preferred surgical approach; denervation with cervical rhizotomy may be also considered in selected patients. The selection of the most effective treatments depends on many factors. However chemodenervation with botulinum toxin is considered the first-line treatment in most clinical settings.

Medical Treatments

Pharmacological treatments include chemodenervation with botulinum toxin injected intramuscularly and oral medications.

Chemodenervation with Botulinum Toxin

Botulinum toxin is a therapeutic agent derived from the anaerobic, gram-positive, rod-shaped bacterium *Clostridium botulinum*. Botulinum toxin comes in many different formulations and has been used effectively for the treatment of cervical dystonia since the early 1980s. Currently three forms of botulinum toxin A are available for treatment of dystonia: onabotulinumtoxin A (Botox), abobotulinumtoxin A (Dysport), and incobotulinumtoxin A (Xeomin), and one form of botulinum toxin B rimabotulinumtoxin B (Myobloc).

Botulinum toxin does not provide a cure but provides symptomatic benefit due to chemodenervation resulting in a decreased release of acetylcholine, the neurotransmitter at the neuromuscular junction required for muscle contraction. This causes reduced activity of the striated or smooth muscle injected. The chemodenervation caused by botulinum toxin is reversible and dose dependant. Botulinum toxin inhibits the docking and opening of the synaptic vesicles, which contain acetylcholine at the presynaptic nerve terminal, and therefore the toxin blocks the neuromuscular transmission.

Botulinum toxin is injected intramuscularly into the neck muscles involved in cervical dystonia and is helpful in relieving the symptoms of cervical dystonia. Identifying the involved muscles could be a challenge due to the changing

TABLE 2.2 Botulinum toxin dosage for individual muscles involved in cervical dystonia in adults

Muscles involved in cervical dystonia	Average dose/units	Number of injection sites
Sternocleidomastoid	50–100	1–4
Scalenus complex	25–50	1–3
Splenius capitis	50–100	1–3
Semispinalis capitis	50–100	1–3
Longissimus capitis	50–75	1–3
Trapezius	50–100	1–4
Levator scapulae	50–100	1–3

The dosing is based on onabotulinumtoxin A (Botox) units. The most common conversion between onabotulinumtoxin A and abobotulinumtoxin A (Dysport) units is 1:2.5, while the units of onabotulinumtoxin A and incobotulinumtoxin A (Xeomin) are exchangeable at 1:1 ratio

pattern of muscle involvement and progression of the conditions. The effect of botulinum toxin becomes apparent within a week after the injections. However, the maximum benefit is reached in 4–6 weeks postinjections and lasts about 10–12 weeks before it starts to wear off and symptoms return. The botulinum toxin injections have to be repeated once the symptoms return.

Botulinum toxin injections are started with a low dosage initially which is adjusted on the subsequent visits (Table 2.2). Excessive doses of botulinum toxin may cause undesired weakness of the treated muscle. Occasionally some patients may find difficulty of swallowing, especially for the first few weeks after injections.

Patients on long-term treatment with botulinum toxin may develop antibodies which would make it ineffective, although this occurs rarely. To check for loss of efficacy, 20 units of botulinum toxin may be injected into the frontalis muscle and reassessed in 2 weeks' time for weakness. No response to botulinum toxin treatment in cervical dystonia may

TABLE 2.3 Medications which may be used drugs in patients with cervical dystonia

Drug	Dosage (mg/day)	Side effects
Trihexyphenidyl (Artane®)	3–15	Dry mouth, confusion, memory problems, bladder dysfunction, and blurred vision
Benztropine (Cogentin®)	1–12	Same as trihexyphenidyl
Clonazepam (Rivotril®)	1–12	Lethargy, sedation, drowsiness
Baclofen (Lioresal®)	20–90	Lethargy, sedation, drowsiness

occur due to many different reasons, the most common being inadequate dosage, inappropriate selection of muscles, dynamic disease change, and rarely development of neutralizing antibodies.

Medications

Anticholinergic medications are the major class of drugs used in cervical dystonia (Table 2.3). Anticholinergic drugs usually show significant beneficial effect at high doses. Children can tolerate the anticholinergic medications better than adults. High doses of anticholinergic medications in the adults are mostly associated with unpleasant side effects. The anticholinergic drugs should be started at a low dosage and titrated slowly. The patients with mild degree of dystonia have better response than those with the severe degree of dystonia; however, the effect of anticholinergic medications may wane over time. The common side effects of anticholinergic medications include dry mouth, confusion, hallucinations, memory problem, urinary bladder dysfunction, and exacerbation of acute-angle glaucoma. The commonly used anticholinergic medications include trihexyphenidyl and benztropine. Muscle relaxants such as lorazepam and baclofen (Lioresal) which is a GABA agonist may be helpful in some cases.

Surgical Treatments of Cervical Dystonia

Presently, surgery is performed only in patients who are refractory to botulinum toxin or medications. Surgical treatment is considered if patients have functional disability or restriction of social activities because of cervical dystonia. Surgical methods can also be used as an additive to conservative treatment in order to reduce drug doses.

Peripheral surgical treatments for cervical dystonia include rhizotomy, selective rhizotomy, and myotomy. Highly selective peripheral denervation surgery ("the Bertrand procedure") reduces the abnormal contraction of the involved muscles by sectioning the nerve supply to these muscles.

Bilateral pallidal deep brain stimulation (DBS) seems promising in patients with severe refractory cervical dystonia. Surgical treatment, combined with several approaches and techniques, can be successfully used in some patients with cervical dystonia.

2.3.9   Neurodegenerative Disorders Associated with Limb Dystonia

The common neurodegenerative disorders associated with limb dystonias, which are usually focal or segmental, include Parkinson's disease, progressive supranuclear palsy, and corticobasal degeneration.

2.3.10   Psychogenic Dystonia

Psychogenic cases are a diagnosis of exclusion. The following features may be helpful in diagnosing psychogenic cases:

1. Abrupt onset of symptoms
2. Abnormal posture or movements disappearing with distraction
3. Inconsistent movements or posture which change characteristics over time

4. Incongruous movements and postures which do not fit the recognized physiological patterns
5. Spontaneous remissions of symptoms
6. Presence of additional abnormal movements not consistent with the basic abnormal movement pattern or not congruous with a known movement disorder such as rhythmical shaking, slowness in carrying out voluntary movement, and excessive startle in response to sudden, unexpected noise or threatening movement
7. Presence of features of a paroxysmal disorder
8. Onset of dystonia with a fixed posture
9. Resolution of symptoms in response to placebo, suggestion, or psychotherapy

Self-inflicted injuries, inconsistent weakness, markedly fluctuating or intermittent dystonia, inconsistent sensory deficit, multiple somatizations or pain, and other abnormal movements, including bizarre gait, are some of the clues which may indicate a possible psychogenic cause of dystonia.

2.3.11   Pseudodystonia

Pseudodystonia may be present with postures similar to cervical dystonia. Pseudodystonias may result from the following conditions:

1. Atlantoaxial subluxation
2. Soft tissue neck mass
3. Syringomyelia
4. Arnold-Chiari malformation
5. Cranial nerve IV palsy
6. Cranial nerve VI palsy
7. Vestibular dysfunction
8. Posterior fossa mass
9. Stiff person syndrome
10. Congenital Klippel-Feil syndrome
11. Sandifer syndrome

Bibliography

Barbanti P, Fabbrini G, Pauletti C, Defazio G, Cruccu G, Berardelli A. Headache in cranial and cervical dystonia. Neurology. 2005;64: 1308–9.

Bereznai B, Steude U, Seelos K, Botzel K. Chronic high-frequency globus pallidus internus stimulation in different types of dystonia: a clinical, video, and MRI report of six patients presenting with segmental, cervical, and generalized dystonia. Mov Disord. 2002;17: 138–44.

Bertrand CM, Molina-Negro P. Selective peripheral denervation in 111 cases of spasmodic torticollis: rationale and results. In: Fahn S, Marsden CD, Calne DB, editors. Dystonia 2, vol. 50. New York: Raven; 1988. p. 637–43.

Bihari K, Hill JL, Murphy DL. Obsessive-compulsive characteristics in patients with idiopathic spasmodic torticollis. Psychiatry Res. 1992;42(3):267–72.

Bradley GW, Daroff R, Fenichel G, Marsden D. Neurology in clinical practice. 5th ed. Butlerworth & Heinmann. Oxford, UK; 2007

Brancati F, Valente EM, Castori M, et al. Role of the dopamine D5 receptor (DRD5) as a susceptibility gene for cervical dystonia. J Neurol Neurosurg Psychiatry. 2003;74:665–6.

Braun V, Richter HP, Schroder JM. Selective peripheral denervation for spasmodic torticollis: is outcome predictable? J Neurol. 1995;242: 504–7.

Chan J, Brin MF, Fahn S. Idiopathic CD: clinical characteristics. Mov Disord. 1991;6:119–26.

Chawda SJ, Munchau A, Johnson D, et al. Pattern of premature degenerative changes of the cervical spine in patients with spasmodic torticollis and the impact on the outcome of selective peripheral denervation. J Neurol Neurosurg Psychiatry. 2000;68:465–71.

Claypool DW, Duane DD, Ilstrup DM, Melton 3rd LJ. Epidemiology and outcome of cervical dystonia (spasmodic torticollis) in Rochester, Minnesota. Mov Disord. 1995;10:608–14.

Clemente CD. Anatomy, a regional atlas of the human body. 3rd ed. Part VI The back, vertebral column and spinal cord. Urban & Schwarzenberg.

Cohen-Gadol AA, Ahlskog JE, Matsumoto JY, Swenson MA, McClelland RL, Davis DH. Selective peripheral denervation for the treatment of intractable spasmodic torticollis: experience with 168 patients at the Mayo Clinic. J Neurosurg. 2003;98:1247–54.

Collins A, Jankovic J. Botulinum toxin injection for congenital muscular torticollis presenting in children and adults. Neurology. 2006;67: 1083–5.

Comella CL, Jankovic J, Shannon KM, et al. Comparison of botulinum toxin serotypes A and B for the treatment of cervical dystonia. Neurology. 2005;65:1423–9.

Dauer WT, Burke RE, Greene P, Fahn S. Current concepts on the clinical features, etiology and management of idiopathic cervical dystonia. Brain. 1998;121:547–60.

Defazio G, Livrea P, Guanti G, Lepore V, Ferrari E. Genetic contribution to idiopathic adult-onset blepharospasm and cranial-cervical dystonia. Eur Neurol. 1993;33:345–50.

Deuschl G, Elble RJ. The pathophysiology of essential tremor. Neurology. 2000;54:S14–20.

Deuschl G, Heinen F, Guschlbauer B, Schneider S, Glocker FX, Lucking CH. Hand tremor in patients with spasmodic torticollis. Mov Disord. 1997;12:547–52.

Duane DD. Spasmodic torticollis: clinical and biological features and their implications for focal dystonia. In: Fahn S, Marsden CD, Calne DB, editors. Dystonia 2, vol. 50. New York: Raven; 1988. p. 473–92.

Dykstra DD, Mendez A, Chappuis D, Baxter T, DesLauriers L, Stuckey M. Treatment of cervical dystonia and focal hand dystonia by high cervical continuously infused intrathecal baclofen: a report of 2 cases. Arch Phys Med Rehabil. 2005;86:830–3.

Fahn S, Bressman S, Marsden CD. Classification of dystonia. Adv Neurol. 1998;78:1–10.

Friedman A, Fahn S. Spontaneous remission in spasmodic torticollis. Neurology. 1986;36:398–400.

Friedman AH, Nashold Jr BS, Sharp R, Caputi F, Arruda J. Treatment of spasmodic torticollis with intradural selective rhizotomies. J Neurosurg. 1993;78:46–53.

Frucht S, Fahn S, Ford B, et al. A geste antagoniste device to treat jaw closing dystonia. Mov Disord. 1999;14:883–6.

Goetz CG, Pappert EJ. Textbook of clinical neurology. 2nd ed. Philadelphia: Saunders; 1999.

Goetz CG, Chmura TA, Lanska DJ. History of dystonia: part 4 history of movement disorders. Mov Disord. 2001;16:339–45.

Greene P, Kang U, Fahn S, Brin M, Moskowitz C, Flaster E. Double-blind, placebo controlled trial of botulinum toxin injections for the treatment of spasmodic torticollis. Neurology. 1990;40:1213–8.

Hung SW, Hamani C, Lozano AM, et al. Long-term outcome of bilateral pallidal deep brain stimulation for primary cervical dystonia. Neurology. 2007;68:457–9.

Huygen PL, Verhagen WI, Van Hoof JJ, Horstink MW. Vestibular hyperactivity in patients with idiopathic spasmodic torticollis. J Neurol Neurosurg Psychiatry. 1989;52:782–5.

Jahanshahi M, Marsden CD. Psychological functioning before and after treatment of torticollis with botulinum toxin. J Neurol Neurosurg Psychiatry. 1992;55:229–31.

Jankovic J. Botulinum toxin in clinical practice. J Neurol Neurosurg Psychiatry. 2004;75:951–7.

Jankovic J, Schwartz K. Botulinum toxin injections for cervical dystonia. Neurology. 1990;40:277–80.

Jankovic J, Tolosa E. Parkinson's disease and movement disorder. 5th ed. Philadelphia: Lippincott Williams and Wilkins; 2007.

Jankovic J, Leder S, Warner D, Schwartz K. Cervical dystonia: clinical findings and associated movement disorders. Neurology. 1991;41: 1088–91.

Jankovic J, Tsui J, Bergeron C. Prevalence of cervical dystonia and spasmodic torticollis in the United States general population. Parkinsonism Relat Disord. 2007;13:411–6.

Kiss ZHT, Doig K, Eliaszi WM, et al. DBS for torticollis: preliminary results from multicenter Canadian pilot study. Can J Neurol Sci. 2004;31 suppl 1:S29.

Koukouni V, Martino D, Arabia G, Quinn NP, Bhatia KP. The entity of young onset primary cervical dystonia. Mov Disord. 2007;22:843–7.

Krauss JK, Loher TJ, Pohle T, et al. Pallidal deep brain stimulation in patients with cervical dystonia and severe cervical dyskinesias with cervical myelopathy. J Neurol Neurosurg Psychiatry. 2002;72:249–56.

Kutvonen O, Dastidar P, Nurmikko T. Pain in spasmodic torticollis. Pain. 1997;69:279–86.

Lew MF, Adornato BT, Duanne DD, et al. Botulinum toxin type B: a double-blind, placebo-controlled, safety and efficacy study in cervical dystonia. Neurology. 1997;49:701–7.

Magyar-Lehmann S, Antonni A, Roelcke U, et al. Cerebral glucose metabolism in patients with spasmodic torticollis. Mov Disord. 1997;12:704–8.

Naumann M, Jankovic J. Safety of botulinum toxin type A: a systematic review and meta-analysis. Curr Med Res Opin. 2004;20:981–90.

Nutt JG, Muenter MD, Joseph III ML, Aronson A, Kurland LT. Epidemiology of dystonia in Rochester, Minnesota. In: Fahn S, Marsden CD, Calne DB, editors. Dystonia 2, vol. 50. New York: Raven; 1988. p. 361–5.

O'Riordan S, Hutchinson M. Cervical dystonia following peripheral trauma – a case–control study. J Neurol. 2004;251:150–5.

Patterson RM, Little SC. Spasmodic torticollis. J Nerv Ment Dis. 1943;98:571–99.

Rana AQ. An introduction to essential tremor. Indiana: iUniverse publishing; 2010.

Ray LW, Koller WC. Movement disorders, neurologic principles and practice. 2nd ed. New York: McGraw-Hill; 1997.

Riski JE, Horner J, Nashold Jr BS. Swallowing function in patients with spasmodic torticollis. Neurology. 1990;40:1443–5.

Rivest J, Marsden CD. Trunk and head tremor as isolated manifestations of dystonia. Mov Disord. 1990;5:60–5.

Rolands LP, editor. Merritt's textbook of neurology. 10th ed. New York: Lippincott Williams & Wilkins; 2000.

Sa DS, Malis-Gagnon A, Nicholson K, Lang AE. Posttraumatic painful torticollis. Mov Disord. 2003;18:1482–91.

Samii A, Pal PK, Schulzer M, Mak E, Tsui JK. Post-traumatic cervical dystonia: a distinct entity? Can J Neurol Sci. 2000;27:55–9.

Schneider S, Feifel E, Ott D, Schumacher M, Lucking CH, Deuschl G. Prolonged MRI T2 times of the lentiform nucleus in idiopathic spasmodic torticollis. Neurology. 1994;44:846–50.

Stemp LI, Taswell C. Spastic torticollis during general anesthesia: case report and review of receptor mechanisms. Anesthesiology. 1991;75:365–6.

Stoessl AJ, Martin WR, Clark C, et al. PET studies of cerebral glucose metabolism in idiopathic torticollis. Neurology. 1986;36:653–7.

Suchowersky O, Calne DB. Non-dystonic causes of torticollis. In: Fahn S, Marsden CD, Calne DB, editors. Dystonia 2, vol. 50. New York: Raven; 1988. p. 501–8.

Sydow O, Thobois S, Alesch F, Speelman JD. Multicentre European study of thalamic stimulation in essential tremor: a six year follow up. J Neurol Neurosurg Psychiatry. 2003;74:1387–91.

Taira T, Hitchcock E. Torticollis as an initial symptom of adult-onset dystonia musculorum deformans. Brain Nerve. 1990;42:867–71.

Tarlov E. On the problem of the pathology of spasmodic torticollis. J Neurol Neurosurg Psychiatry. 1970;33:457–63.

Tolosa E, Montserrat L, Bayes A. Blink reflex studies in focal dystonias: enhanced excitability of brainstem interneurons in cranial dystonia and spasmodic torticollis. Mov Disord. 1988;3:61–9.

Truong DD, Dubinsky R, Hermanowicz N, Olson WL, Silverman B, Koller WC. Posttraumatic torticollis. Arch Neurol. 1991;48:221–3.

Tsui JK, Stoessl AJ, Eisen A, Calne S, Calne DB. Double-blind study of botulinum toxin in spasmodic torticollis. Lancet. 1986;8501:245–7.

Uitti RJ, Maraganore DM. Adult onset familial cervical dystonia: report of a family including monozygotic twins. Mov Disord. 1993;8:489–94.

Waddy HM, Fletcher NA, Harding AE, Marsden CD. A genetic study of idiopathic focal dystonias. Ann Neurol. 1991;29:320–4.

Yianni J, Bain P, Giladi N, et al. Globus pallidus internus deep brain stimulation for dystonic conditions: a prospective audit. Mov Disord. 2003;18:436–42.

Chapter 3
Chorea

Abstract   Chorea is characterized by involuntary, brief, unpredictable, and random hyperkinetic movements. This chapter reviews main clinical characteristics of chorea and similar hyperkinetic movements and their most common causes. We describe characteristic phenotypic features of chorea-causing conditions, their differential diagnosis, and most useful clinical work-up, including genetic testing. We also discuss most typical clinical presentation of the most common types of chorea, especially Huntington's disease with its motor and non-motor symptoms and signs, and main therapeutic options. Additional emphasis is on treatable causes of chorea, such as Sydenham chorea and Wilson's disease.

Keywords   Chorea • Huntington's disease • Therapy • Hyperkinetic movements • Tetrabenazine

Chorea is characterized by involuntary, brief, unpredictable, fleeing movements which may seem to flow from one body part to another randomly. When these movements are slower and more flowing, they may be referred as *athetosis*, whereas when choreic movements are more severe, they are referred to as *ballism*. These movements may convey to the observer an impression of restlessness of the affected individual.

A.Q. Rana, P. Hedera, *Differential Diagnosis of Movement Disorders in Clinical Practice*, DOI 10.1007/978-3-319-01607-8_3, © Springer International Publishing Switzerland 2014

3.1   Classification

Chorea can be classified into two groups: nongenetic and genetic chorea. Nongenetic causes of chorea include vascular causes, Sydenham and other autoimmune chorea, drug-induced causes, metabolic causes, and infections. The common genetic causes of chorea include Huntington's disease, whereas the rare causes include neuroacanthocytosis, McLoed syndrome, benign hereditary chorea, and Wilson's disease.

3.2   Investigations

History and detailed neurological examination is important in the assessment of chorea. Genetic testing and imaging of brain may be required in some cases. Other serological investigations which may be helpful include ANA, CBC with peripheral smear examination for acanthocytes, antiphospholipid antibodies, and lupus anticoagulant.

Although elevated antistreptolysin-O titer may be found in patients with Sydenham chorea, it may also be elevated in groups with a high occurrence of streptococcal infection. Moreover, the antistreptolysin-O titer declines if the time period between infection and rheumatic fever is greater than several weeks. Doppler echocardiography is important due to the common link of Sydenham chorea with carditis.

The diagnosis of Wilson's disease is normally based on the distinctive biochemical abnormalities such as elevated urine copper, low serum ceruloplasmin, and the identification of the Kayser-Fleischer rings. Other investigations may be directed to the suspected underlying causes.

3.3   Differential Diagnosis of Phenomenology of Chorea

What distinguishes chorea from tremor and dystonia is its unpredictable nature. Tremor is characterized by rhythmic contractions of antagonist muscles. On the other hand, the universal sign of dystonia is the rhythmic contraction of muscles resulting in abnormal postures or torsional movements.

Chorea sometimes gets confused with tics. Tics can be easily differentiated from chorea because they reproduce normal human vocalizations/movements and are usually preceded by a local unpleasant sensation. Tics can also be voluntarily suppressed, whereas chorea cannot.

Athetosis illustrates slow, flowing movements affecting distal limbs, especially in the arms. The term athetosis is slowly being abandoned in medical literature due to the reason that it is better defined as dystonia related with some degree of chorea.

The term athetosis has been used previously to describe the combination of chorea and dystonia in the distal portions of limbs in individuals affected by cerebral palsy. Even though athetosis was traditionally illustrated as a complication of kernicterus, it may occur in cerebral palsy of any cause. The phenomenology of athetosis is described by a variable combination of myoclonus, spasticity, dystonia, and chorea. The pseudoathetosis describes slow, distal writhing movements of the fingers or toes in patients with proprioceptive loss and is illustrated in accordance with peripheral neuropathy. It should be noted, however, that pseudoathetosis can also be caused by central lesions resulting in impairment of proprioception (thalamic lesion, myelopathy, or others).

3.4 Causes

3.4.1 Genetic Causes of Chorea

Huntington's Disease

Huntington's disease is a neurodegenerative condition transmitted in an autosomal dominant fashion. The onset is usually in midlife and the symptoms progress over several years.

Huntington's disease is a rare condition with a prevalence of 5–10 individuals per 100,000 in Europe. In Japan, Huntington's disease is extremely rare, with a prevalence of less than 0.5 per 100,000.

Initially patient may develop anxiety, behavioral changes, sleep disturbances, depression, general restlessness, and hygienic neglect. Motor signs usually appear after but can occur at the onset of the disease and include involuntary movements which cannot be suppressed by the patient. The characteristic facial movements and postures include raising eyebrows, leading to the facial expression of an astonished appearance. Patients have clumsiness upon rapid alternating hand movements or finger tapping. Uncontrolled finger and truncal movements are also apparent. The chorea usually exacerbates during stress, walking, and concentration. Most patients are more aware of their mood swings than choreiform movements.

With the evolution of the disease, chorea becomes worse and impairs voluntary movements and gait balance. Rigidity and bradykinesia are common in juvenile cases where chorea may be absent. Dystonic postures of the limbs, trunk, and neck are common. Gait and motor speed are both affected with the increasing risk of falls. In some cases, there is evidence of cerebellar dysfunction, and eye movements are always abnormal. Individuals generally have trouble initiating saccades and decrease in saccade velocity. The eye movement abnormalities can be seen in presymptomatic stages.

Patients usually have hyperreflexia with extensor plantar responses, and dysarthria is frequent, and speech disturbance is usually mixed, occasionally cerebellar in nature. Weight loss and sleep disturbances are also common.

As the condition advances, motor disability becomes severe, the patient becoming incontinent and dependent upon others for activities of daily life. The average survival time after the diagnoses of HD usually varies from 5 to 30 years.

Behavior disorders differentiate Huntington's disease from other causes of chorea. Patients usually have anxiety that can be disabling and accompanied with depression. In early stages, patients have decreased mood, loss of energy, interest, and appetite. With the progression of disease, patients may develop impulsivity, irritability, and untreated anxiety which can lead to violent and aggressive behavior.

Low self-esteem with feelings of hopelessness is not uncommon, and the risk of suicide is also increased. The psychiatric symptoms respond well to pharmacological treatment.

Cognitive changes may be present in the early stages of Huntington's disease and may precede motor symptoms and depression. The usual cognitive changes include reduced mental flexibility, memory problems, impaired working memory, and slowness of execution. Planning and organization of sequential activities affects everyday tasks. Decreased attention capacities and global inertia with subcortical dementia are frequent.

The diagnosis of Huntington's disease can be established clinically due to the presence of affective and cognitive changes associated with progressive motor dysfunction, family history consistent with autosomal dominant transmission, and behavioral problems.

The diagnosis of Huntington's disease is supported by the atrophy of the caudate nucleus, although MRI is used more commonly to rule out other neurological conditions. Pathologic studies show severe and progressive atrophy of the putamen and caudate. Proteins with lengthened polyglutamine tracts aggregate to form intraneuronal inclusions and may appear before other symptoms of disease.

The HD gene mutation with trinucleotide CAG repeat expansion is the main gene abnormality in Huntington's disease. The HDL2 gene mutation is a rare gene abnormality causing Huntington's disease with similar phenotype.

For an extensive period of time, Huntington's disease was considered a genetically homogenous disorder with a single gene (HD gene or IT15) mutation on chromosome 4p, leading to CAG repeat expansion. Although this mutation is responsible for the vast majority of cases of Huntington's disease, presently genetic heterogeneity is known due to mutation involving Junctophilin 3 gene or HDL2 gene, causing a typical Huntington's disease phenotype in a small number of patients.

Juvenile Huntington's disease is considered with onset before the age of 21 and is responsible for nearly 5–15 % of all Huntington's disease cases. In majority of cases the transmission of juvenile Huntington's disease is paternal, and the number of CAG repeats in the HD gene is larger than 60. Maternal transmission of juvenile Huntington's disease with abnormally large expansions has also been reported. These patients have seizures and prominent rigidity with dystonia, while the chorea is minimal.

Huntington's disease gene is located on chromosome 4p16.3 with CAG trinucleotide repeat above the threshold of 36 in a heterozygous state in individuals. Individuals with 36–38 CAG repeats have a reduced penetrance and may not exhibit HD during a regular life-span. In many cases the size of the expansion increases even more during transmission, resulting in an average increase of the expansion size in successive generations. Paternal transmissions are associated with the greatest tendency to increase in size and instability. There are also intermediate sizes of repeats which range from 27 to 35, although not linked with the disease, but are commonly susceptible to expansion, even if the estimated risk is very rare. However, very few patients with CAG repeats falling within the intermediate allele size develop clinical signs of HD. Intermediate alleles can also display instability during paternal transmissions, which indicates that the offspring of a male intermediate allele carrier risks the inheritance of a larger allele which can be linked to Huntington's disease. On the contrary, no expansion of intermediate alleles has been observed maternally. Although the abnormal repeat size varies from 36 to 200 units, alleles with 40 to 45 repeats are predominant in most patients affected with Huntington's disease.

Huntington's disease was originally believed to be monogenetic with one responsible gene and one single mutation in the HD gene. However, the association of HDL2 or Junctophilin 3 located on chromosome 1 6q confirmed genetic heterogeneity in Huntington's disease. The observed mutation is an expanded CAG repeat, which varies from 44 to 57 repeats. HDL2 gene may be more common in populations from black African ancestry. Several patients with HDL2 have prominent hypokinetic syndrome, thus resembling a juvenile form of HD.

Management

A multidisciplinary approach is essential in managing Huntington's disease. Depression, anxiety, cognitive dysfunction, and chorea each should be managed individually. Neuroleptics and atypical antipsychotics—such as quetiapine, olanzapine without sedation, and clozapine—may be used when required. Early treatment may lead to better compliance. Since antichoreic therapy may have potential side effects, chorea is only treated if patients are bothered or if gait is affected.

Tetrabenazine helps chorea but may result in depression. There is variable evidence that L-dopa improves rigidity and bradykinesia. Physical therapy with a focus on balance and gait training may help implications of chorea. Speech therapy may provide some help in improving communication strategies.

Selective serotonin reuptake inhibitors (SSRIs) are helpful for depression. They may provide some relief to anxiety, although obsessive-compulsive symptoms respond better to atypical neuroleptics.

Dentatorubropallidoluysian Atrophy (DRPLA)

Dentatorubropallidoluysian atrophy is transmitted in an autosomal dominant fashion with anticipation responsible for the differences in juvenile- and adult-onset cases. The genetic defect is trinucleotide repeat of CAG located on chromosome 12p, causing mutations in a protein called atrophin-1. It is a rare condition and initial cases were described from Japan, but other families from North America and Europe have been reported as well. There is neuronal loss and gliosis in the dentate nucleus, red nucleus, external globus pallidus, and subthalamic nucleus. There is diversity in the phenotype including chorea, myoclonus, seizures, cerebellar ataxia, and dementia.

Neuroacanthocytosis

Neuroacanthocytosis is characterized by cognitive dysfunction, movement disorder such as chorea, and behavioral changes. The gene for neuroacanthocytosis is located on chromosome 9q21. Although neuroacanthocytosis is an autosomal recessively transmitted condition, as well, some families are affected by autosomal dominant forms of inheritance. Amyotrophy and areflexia are frequent and nerve conduction studies may show peripheral neuropathy. More than half of individuals affected by neuroacanthocytosis have a self-mutilating oro-mandibulo-lingual dystonia which involves biting of the tongue. Tonic-clonic generalized seizures are not uncommon and some patients may have vocal tics as well. There may be increased serum level of creatine kinase, and about 10 % or more of the peripheral red cells in patients with neuroacanthocytosis consist of acanthocytes although this level may vary as the disease progresses. Parkinsonism can be the sole movement disorder in neuroacanthocytosis, whereas in Huntington's disease this is not the case.

McLeod Syndrome

The clinical features of McLeod syndrome can be difficult to differentiate from neuroacanthocytosis. Self-mutilating tongue dystonia and seizures are frequent in patients affected by neuroacanthocytosis, whereas more patients with McLeod syndrome have cardiomyopathy and myopathy. McLeod syndrome and neuroacanthocytosis can however both be accurately distinguished by observing the gene CHAC in neuroacanthocytosis and the low reactivity of Kell erythrocyte antigens, the universal sign of McLeod syndrome. Patients with McLeod syndrome with seizure disorder may require antiepileptic drugs as valproic acid or carbamazepine. For self-mutilating lingual dystonia, botulinum toxin is considered an effective treatment.

Benign Hereditary Chorea

The clinical features of benign hereditary chorea manifest before the age of 5 years and include chorea, autosomal dominant transmission, and ataxia in minority of the patients. Their course may be static or with spontaneous improvement after childhood. After the discovery of a mutation of the TITF-1 gene mutation on chromosome 14q, it is considered independent nosologic entity.

Wilson's Disease

The neurological signs of this rare autosomal recessive condition are caused by a mutation in the ATP7B gene on chromosome 13q. This condition results in deposition of copper in the brain, predominantly in the upper brainstem and basal ganglia. Because Wilson's disease can be treated effectively with agents that chelate copper and prevent its absorption, it should be included in differential diagnosis of patients of 40 years of age or younger with movement disorders. A fatal outcome is associated with cases of Wilson's disease, if left untreated. The clinical phenotype of Wilson's disease is rather varied, with chorea, tremor, parkinsonism, and dystonia. It should be noted, however, that isolated chorea is seldom observed in these patients. The diagnosis of Wilson's disease is normally based on the distinctive biochemical abnormalities such as elevated urine copper, low serum ceruloplasmin, and the identification of the Kayser-Fleischer rings.

3.4.2   Nongenetic Causes of Chorea

Sydenham Chorea

Sydenham chorea is an autoimmune condition occurring in approximately one fourth of patients with rheumatic fever. Despite its declining incidence, Sydenham chorea remains one of the most frequent causes of acute chorea in children worldwide.

The usual age of onset of Sydenham chorea is around 8 years, although there have been reports of individuals developing Sydenham chorea in their 30s. Sydenham chorea is rarely seen before the age of 5 years. Usually, patients develop choreiform movements a few weeks after an episode of group A β-hemolytic streptococcus (GABHS) pharyngitis. In some cases, although choreiform movements may become generalized, in one fifth of patients, it is localized to one side of body. Individuals affected with Sydenham chorea show motor impersistence, particularly noticeable during ocular fixation and tongue protrusion. These patients may have decreased muscle tone, in rare cases making patients bedridden as a result.

Choreiform movements in patients with Sydenham chorea may be difficult to differentiate from simple tics. Vocal tics may be found in some patients with Sydenham chorea, the exact cause of which is unclear.

Peripheral nervous system is believed not to be involved in Sydenham chorea. Sydenham chorea is a major manifestation of rheumatic fever. More than two thirds of patients with Sydenham chorea exhibit cardiac involvement, especially mitral valve dysfunction. The association of Sydenham chorea with arthritis is less common and may be observed in one third of the patients.

The pathogenesis of Sydenham chorea is believed to be due to existence of molecular imitation between central nervous system and streptococcal antigens. Group A β-hemolytic streptococcal infection in genetically predisposed patients leads to the formation of antibodies which are cross-reactive with the basal ganglia. Numerous studies have shown the presence of such circulating antibodies in more than half of the individuals with Sydenham chorea.

The current criteria for the diagnosis of Sydenham chorea include chorea with lack of evidence of alternative causes of chorea. The diagnosis is supported even further by the presence of additional minor or major signs of rheumatic fever. The goal of the diagnostic work-up in patients suspected to be affected with Sydenham chorea is to rule out alternative causes of Sydenham chorea, identify evidence of recent streptococcal infection or acute phase reaction in the individual affected with SC, and rule out any cardiac injury associated with rheumatic fever.

Investigations such as C-reactive protein, leukocytosis, erythrocyte sedimentation rate, and other blood tests such as protein electrophoresis, rheumatoid factor, mucoproteins, and supporting evidence of preceding streptococcal infection (such as increased antiDNAse-B, antistreptolysin-O, and positive throat culture for group A *Streptococcus*) are usually not helpful in Sydenham chorea than in other forms of rheumatic fever because of the generally lengthy latency between the infection and onset of the chorea.

An elevated antistreptolysin-O titer may be found in groups with a high occurrence of streptococcal infection. Moreover, the antistreptolysin-O titer declines if the time period between infection and rheumatic fever is greater than several weeks. Doppler echocardiography is important due to the common link of Sydenham chorea with carditis. Normally, neuroimaging will help to rule out structural causes of chorea. A CT scan of the brain is usually not helpful. MRI of the head is also usually normal, although there are reports of reversible hyperintensity in the basal ganglia.

Sydenham chorea is usually a self-limited condition that may go in remission after a course of 8–9 months. Valproic acid is the commonly used medication, although other anticonvulsants such as carbamazepine are also effective. Dopamine receptor-blocking agents, such as pimozide, are generally used in patients who fail to respond to the abovementioned medications.

The role of immunosuppression in the management of Sydenham chorea is controversial. Steroids are often reserved for patients with chorea resistant to other treatments. There are some reports of use of intravenous immunoglobulin or plasma exchange in the treatment of Sydenham chorea. Secondary prophylaxis with penicillin or sulfa drugs is important up to the age of 21.

There have been reports of half of the patients remaining with chorea up to 2 years. Despite the use of secondary prophylaxis, recurrences of Sydenham chorea may be observed in almost half of the cases.

Vascular Chorea

Vascular chorea may be a rare complication of acute stroke in less than 1 % of patients. The resulting movement which is often regarded as *hemiballism* is generally related to hemorrhagic or ischemic lesion of the basal ganglia. Although vascular chorea usually goes in remission spontaneously, in the acute phase patients may need treatment with dopamine-depleting drugs. A small number of patients with vascular chorea may also develop persistent choreiform movements. These individuals may require surgical treatments for chorea.

Other rare causes of vascular chorea include Moyamoya disease and post-pump chorea which is a complication of extracorporeal circulation. The etiology of post-pump chorea is vascular insult of the basal ganglia during surgery; however, the course of post-pump chorea is benign with complete remission in most patients.

Other Autoimmune Chorea

Additional rare immunologic causes of chorea are vasculitis, paraneoplastic syndromes, and systemic lupus erythematosus. However, many reports display that chorea is seen in no more than 1–2 % of patients with these conditions.

Drug-Induced Chorea

Chorea may be drug induced; particularly prolonged use of dopamine-blocking drugs may cause chorea. Levodopa-induced chorea is the most common form of drug-induced chorea, although there are some reports of chorea due to other drugs such as lamotrigine or lithium. Chorea usually resolves after discontinuation of these drugs. Other drugs which may cause chorea include neuroleptics, anticholinergics, calcium channel blockers, cocaine, amphetamine, SSRIs such as fluoxetine, and tricyclic antidepressants including imipramine. Oral contraceptive-induced chorea and chorea gravidarum, or chorea occurring during pregnancy, are thought to have similar mechanism.

Chorea Due to Metabolic Causes

Chorea due to nonketotic hyperglycemia occurs mainly in type II diabetes mellitus. These patients do not develop changes in levels of consciousness but do develop generalized or unilateral chorea ballism. The MRI may show characteristic hyperintense signal in the pallidum on T1. After adequate glycemic control is attained, there is a steady remission of chorea.

Acquired hepatolenticular degeneration was the first well-described metabolic cause of chorea. These patients have asterixis, somnolence, myoclonus, tremor, chorea, apathy, and parkinsonism.

A small number of patients with hyperthyroidism may develop generalized chorea or even ballism. Other possible metabolic causes of chorea may include renal failure, ketogenic diet, and hypoglycemia.

Chorea Due to Infectious Causes

HIV and its complications have comprised the most frequently reported infectious cause of chorea. In HIV-positive patients, the direct action of the virus or other mechanisms, such as opportunistic infections (syphilis, toxoplasmosis, and others) or drugs, resulted in chorea. Other infections related to chorea are tuberculosis and the new variant Creutzfeldt-Jakob disease.

Bibliography

Asherson RA, Cervera R. Unusual manifestations of the antiphospholipid syndrome. Clin Rev Allergy Immunol. 2003;25:61–78.

Bader B, Vollmar C, Ackl N, Ebert A, la Fougère C, Noachtar S, Danek A. Bilateral temporal lobe epilepsy confirmed with intracranial EEG in chorea-acanthocytosis. Seizure. 2011;20:340–2.

Baizabal-Carvallo JF, Alonso-Juarez M, Koslowski M. Chorea in systemic lupus erythematosus. J Clin Rheumatol. 2011;17:69–72.

Breedveld GJ, Percy AK, MacDonald ME, et al. Clinical and genetic heterogeneity in benign hereditary chorea. Neurology. 2002;59:579–84.

Brilot F, Merheb V, Ding A, Murphy T, Dale RC. Antibody binding to neuronal surface in Sydenham chorea, but not in PANDAS or Tourette syndrome. Neurology. 2011;76:1508–13.

Cardoso F. Chorea gravidarum. Arch Neurol. 2002;59:868–70.

Cardoso F. Sydenham's chorea. Handb Clin Neurol. 2011;100:221–9.

Cardoso F, Maia D, Cunningham MC, Valenca G. Treatment of Sydenham chorea with corticosteroids. Mov Disord. 2003;18:1374–7.

Carroll E, Sanchez-Ramos J. Hyperkinetic movement disorders associated with HIV and other viral infections. Handb Clin Neurol. 2011;100: 323–34.

Cortese I, Chaudhry V, So YT, Cantor F, Cornblath DR, Rae-Grant A. Evidence-based guideline update: plasmapheresis in neurologic disorders: report of the Therapeutics and Technology Assessment Subcommittee of the American Academy of Neurology. Neurology. 2011;76:294–300.

Cummins A, Eggert J, Pruitt R, Collins JS. Huntington disease: implications for practice. Nurse Pract. 2011;36:41–7.

Dale RC, Yin K, Ding A, et al. Antibody binding to neuronal surface in movement disorders associated with lupus and antiphospholipid antibodies. Dev Med Child Neurol. 2011;53:522–8.

de Tommaso M, Serpino C, Sciruicchio V. Management of Huntington's disease: role of tetrabenazine. Ther Clin Risk Manag. 2011;7:123–9.

Docherty MJ, Burn DJ. Hyperthyroid chorea. Handb Clin Neurol. 2011;100:279–86.

Eidelberg D, Surmeier DJ. Brain networks in Huntington disease. J Clin Invest. 2011;121:484–92.

Em JJ, Chang MK. Hemiballism-hemichorea and non-ketotic hyperglycaemia. J Neurol Neurosurg Psychiatry. 1994;57:748–50.

Goetz CG, Pappert EJ. Textbook of clinical neurology. 2nd ed. Philadelphia: Saunders; 1999.

Hagiwara K, Tominaga K, Okada Y, et al. Post-streptococcal chorea in an adult with bilateral striatal encephalitis. J Clin Neurosci. 2011;18:708–9.

Ikeuchi T, Koide R, Onodera O, et al. Dentatorubral – pallidoluysian atrophy (DRPLA): molecular basis for wide clinical features of DRPLA. Clin Neurosci. 1995;3:23–7.

Illarioshkin SN, Igarashi S, Onodera O, et al. Trinucleotide repeat length and rate of progression of Huntington's disease. Ann Neurol. 1994;36: 630–5.

Inzelberg R, Weinberger M, Gak E. Benign hereditary chorea: an update. Parkinsonism Relat Disord. 2011;17:301–7.

Ishaq S, Khalil S, Khan A, Khalid U. Chorea as an unusual presenting feature of anti-phospholipid syndrome. J Pak Med Assoc. 2010;60:975–6.

Jankovic J, Tolosa E. Parkinson's disease and movement disorder. 5th ed. Philadelphia: Lippincott Williams and Wilkins; 2007.

Johri A, Chaturvedi RK, Beal MF. Hugging tight in Huntington's. Nat Med. 2011;17:245–6.

Kimber TE, Thompson PD. Senile chorea. Handb Clin Neurol. 2011; 100:213–7.

Kleiner-Fisman G. Benign hereditary chorea. Handb Clin Neurol. 2011; 100:199–212.

Klempíř J, Zidovská J, Stochl J, Ing VK, Uhrová T, Roth J. The number of CAG repeats within the normal allele does not influence the age of onset in Huntington's disease. Mov Disord. 2011;26:125–9.

Kobayashi K, Aoyama N, Sasaki J, et al. MRI appearance of a cerebral cavernous malformation in the caudate nucleus before and after chorea onset. J Clin Neurosci. 2011;18:719–21.

Kremer HP. Imaging Huntington's disease (HD) brains – imagine HD trails. Neurol Neurosurg Psychiatry. 2005;76:620.

Kremer B, Goldberg P, Andrew SE, et al. A worldwide study of the Huntington's disease mutation. The sensitivity and specificity of measuring CAG repeats. N Engl J Med. 1994;330:1401–6.

Kuehn BM. Imaging helps to identify early changes associated with Huntington disease. JAMA. 2011;305:138.

Le Ber I, Camuzat A, Castelnova G, et al. Prevalence of dentatorubral pallidoluysian atrophy in a large series of white patients with cerebellar ataxia. Arch Neurol. 2003;60:1097–9.

Leung JG, Breden EL. Tetrabenazine for the treatment of tardive dyskinesia. Ann Pharmacother. 2011;45:525–31.

Lewin AB, Storch EA, Murphy TK. Pediatric autoimmune neuropsychiatric disorders associated with Streptococcus in identical siblings. J Child Adolesc Psychopharmacol. 2011;21:177–82.

Marder K, Zhao H, Myers RH, et al. Rate of functional decline in Huntington's disease. Neurology. 2000;54:452–8.

Margolis RL, Homes SE, Rosenblatt A, et al. Huntington's disease like 2 (HDL2) in North America and Japan. Ann Neurol. 2004;56:670–4.

Marshall FJ. A randomized, double blind placebo-controlled study of tetrabenazine in patients with Huntington's disease. Mov Disord. 2004;19:1122.

Marvi MM, Lew MF. Polycythemia and chorea. Handb Clin Neurol. 2011;100:271–6.

Miyasaki JM. Chorea caused by toxins. Handb Clin Neurol. 2011;100:335–46.

Mochel F, Haller RG. Energy deficit in Huntington disease: why it matters. J Clin Invest. 2011;121:493–9.

Ondo WG. Hyperglycemic nonketotic states and other metabolic imbalances. Handb Clin Neurol. 2011;100:287–91.

Paulsen JS, Ready RE, Hamilton JM, Mega MS, Cummings JL. Neuropsychiatric aspects of Huntington's disease. J Neurol Neurosurg Psychiatry. 2001;71:310–4.

Paulsen JS, Hoth KF, Nehl C, Stierman L. Critical periods of suicide risk in Huntington's disease. Am J Psychiatry. 2005;162:725–31.

Perlman SL. Spinocerebellar degenerations. Handb Clin Neurol. 2011;100:113–40.

Piccolo I, Defanti CA, Soliveri P, et al. Cause and course in a series of patients with sporadic chorea. J Neurol. 2003;250:429–35.

Przekop A, Sanger TD. Birth-related syndromes of athetosis and kernicterus. Handb Clin Neurol. 2011;100:387–95.

Przekop A, McClure C, Ashwal S. Postoperative encephalopathy with choreoathetosis. Handb Clin Neurol. 2011;100:295–305.

Ray LW, Koller WC. Movement disorders, neurologic principles and practice. 2nd ed. New York: McGraw-Hill; 1997.

Reglodi D, Kiss P, Lubics A, Tamas A. Review on the protective effects of PACAP in models of neurodegenerative diseases in vitro and in vivo. Curr Pharm Des. 2011;17:962–72.

Robottom BJ, Weiner WJ. Chorea gravidarum. Handb Clin Neurol. 2011;100:231–5.

Rolands LP, editor. Merritt's textbook of neurology. 10th ed. New York: Lippincott Williams & Wilkins; 2000.

Rozas JL, Gómez-Sánchez L, Tomás-Zapico C, Lucas JJ, Fernández-Chacón R. Increased neurotransmitter release at the neuromuscular junction in a mouse model of polyglutamine disease. J Neurosci. 2011;31:1106–13.

Sadeghian H, O'Suilleabhain PE, Battiste J, Elliott JL, Trivedi JR. Huntington chorea presenting with motor neuron disease. Arch Neurol. 2011;68:650–2.

Sah DW, Aronin N. Oligonucleotide therapeutic approaches for Huntington disease. J Clin Invest. 2011;121:500–7.

Schneider SA, Bhatia KP. Huntington's disease look-alikes. Handb Clin Neurol. 2011;100:101–12.

Shirendeb U, Reddy AP, Manczak M, et al. Abnormal mitochondrial dynamics, mitochondrial loss and mutant huntingtin oligomers in Huntington's disease: implications for selective neuronal damage. Hum Mol Genet. 2011;20:1438–55.

Stemper B, Thurauf N, Neundorfer B, Heckmann JG. Choreoathetosis related to lithium intoxication. Eur J Neurol. 2003;10:743–4.

Stevanin G, Fujigasaki H, Lebre AS, et al. Huntington's disease like phenotype due to trinucleotide repeat expansions in the TBP and JPH3 genes. Brain. 2003;126:1599–603.

Tani LY, Veasy LG, Minich LL, Shaddy RE. Rheumatic fever in children younger than 5 years; is the presentation different? Pediatrics. 2003;112:1065–8.

Thobois S, Bozio A, Ninet J, Akhavi A, Broussolle E. Chorea after cardiopulmonary bypass. Eur Neurol. 2004;51:46–7.

Walker HK. An overview of the nervous system. In: Walker HK, Hall WD, Hurst JW, editors. Clinical methods: the history, physical, and laboratory examinations. 3rd ed. Boston: Butterworths; 1990a. Chapter 50.

Walker HK. Involuntary movements. In: Walker HK, Hall WD, Hurst JW, editors. Clinical methods: the history, physical, and laboratory examinations. 3rd ed. Boston: Butterworths; 1990b. Chapter 70.

Walker RH, Rasmussen A, Rudnicki D, et al. Huntington's disease like 2 can present as chorea acanthocytosis. Neurology. 2003;61:1002–4.

Walker RH, Jung HH, Danek A. Neuroacanthocytosis. Handb Clin Neurol. 2011;100:141–51.

Walterfang M, Evans A, Looi JC, et al. The neuropsychiatry of neuroacanthocytosis syndromes. Neurosci Biobehav Rev. 2011a;35:1275–83.

Walterfang M, Looi JC, Styner M, et al. Shape alterations in the striatum in chorea-acanthocytosis. Psychiatry Res. 2011b;192:29–36.

Zesiewicz TA, Sullivan KL. Drug-induced hyperkinetic movement disorders by nonneuroleptic agents. Handb Clin Neurol. 2011;100: 347–63.

Zijlmans JC. Vascular chorea in adults and children. Handb Clin Neurol. 2011;100:261–70.

Chapter 4
Tics

Abstract Tics are sudden, nonrhythmic, repetitive, stereotyped motor movements that are temporarily suppressible and may resemble purposeful-like movements. This chapter reviews main clinical characteristics of ticks and their most common causes. We describe characteristic phenotypic features of conditions associated with both motor and vocal ticks, their differential diagnosis, and most useful clinical work-up. The main emphasis is on Tourette syndrome and its clinical management, including motor and non-motor presentation of this common neurologic condition.

Keywords Tics • Hyperkinetic movements • Tourette syndrome • Obsessive-compulsive disorder

A tic is a sudden, nonrhythmic, repetitive, stereotyped motor movement or vocalization involving discrete muscle groups.

4.1 Classification

There are two main clinical types of tics, which include *motor tics* and *vocal tics*. Motor tics can be simple and complex. Simple motor tics can be further classified as clonic and dystonic. Similarly, vocal tics can be simple or complex.

A.Q. Rana, P. Hedera, *Differential Diagnosis of Movement Disorders in Clinical Practice*, DOI 10.1007/978-3-319-01607-8_4,
© Springer International Publishing Switzerland 2014

Some of the examples of simple motor tics include eye blinking, eyebrow raising, and facial grimacing, whereas complex motor tics include head jerking and jumping. Simple vocal tics include sniffing and throat clearing, whereas complex vocal tics include coprolalia and whistling. Tics are regarded as the universal clinical sign of Tourette syndrome.

4.2   General Presentations

As mentioned above, tics may be simple or complex. Simple motor tics are short, jerk-like movements which are sudden in onset and rapid, such as *clonic tics*, e.g., blinking and head jerking. However, they may also be slower and cause a brief abnormal posturing, such as *dystonic tics*, e.g., sustained mouth opening, bruxism, and shoulder rotation.

Most of the patients with motor and phonic tics have preceding premonitory sensations such as tension or burning feeling in the eye before a blink.

Complex motor tics consist of sequenced and coordinated movements that resemble normal acts that are inappropriately intense. On the contrary, simple phonic tics normally consist of squeaking, grunting, sniffing, throat clearing, blowing, screaming, coughing, and sucking sounds. Tics can typically be volitionally suppressed, but it may require an intense mental effort. Besides temporary suppressibility, tics are also characterized by exacerbation and suggestibility with stress, fatigue, and excitement. Tics may increase while relaxing after a period of stress.

Although tics usually can be suppressed for short periods of time, the inner sensation builds up, consequently leading to a burst of tics when the patient stops suppressing them. Tics usually begin in the neck (head shaking) and face (grimacing, eye blinking). They may spread to further involve the limbs and may be accompanied by various sounds (barking, throat clearing, sniffing, words, or parts of words) and sometimes by foul utterances (coprolalia). Repeating movements (echopraxia) or sounds (echolalia) are often observed.

Simple clonic tics can resemble essential myoclonus, which makes it extremely difficult to distinguish between the two conditions. Dystonic tics should be differentiated from primary torsion dystonia. Intermittency, suppressibility, and premonitory sensations help distinguish tics from most other movement disorders.

Generally, tics start around age 5–6 years and increase in intensity, reaching its most severe period at around age 10. After age 10, there is generally a steady decline in the severity of the disorder. By the age of 18 years, about half of all patients are virtually free from tics.

4.3 Investigations

Usually no investigations are required in majority of patients with tics.

4.4 Causes

4.4.1 Tourette Syndrome

The Gilles de la Tourette syndrome, generally shortened to *Tourette syndrome*, is characterized by both phonic and multiple motor tics that change in character over time, with onset before 21 years of age and symptoms that wane and wax but last more than a year. It is considered the most common cause of tics.

Although the definition is a helpful criterion for research on the disorder, it excludes chronic motor tics or an onset beyond the age of 21 years. It is possible that these conditions may represent milder expressions of Tourette syndrome.

Although it was once considered a rare psychiatric condition, Tourette syndrome is now regarded as a relatively general and intricate neurologic condition. The prevalence of Tourette syndrome in adolescents is around 5 per 10,000 in males and 3 per 10,000 in females.

Several patients have a behavioral component of obsessive-compulsive or attention-deficit disorder. Tourette syndrome may also be associated with hyperactive behavior. The genetic inheritance pattern of Tourette syndrome is controversial.

In patients who have come to necropsy, no specific morphologic changes in the brain have been observed. Dopamine receptors are not increased in the striatum, but hyperinnervation with dopamine terminals has been taken into account by increased mazindol binding. Neuroimaging has displayed incoherent asymmetries in the basal ganglia, in which serum antibodies against the putamen have been found.

When tics are mild and not socially disabling, no treatment is required. However, when more severe, motor and phonic tics can sometimes be reduced with clonazepam and clonidine. Dopamine depletors and antagonists are most effective in the treatment of tics. Pimozide (Orap®) is indicated for the suppression of motor and phonic tics in patients with Tourette syndrome who have failed to respond satisfactorily to standard treatment. It is not intended as a treatment of first choice nor is it intended for the treatment of tics that are merely cosmetically troublesome. Other classic neuroleptics can be also used and the patients must be monitored for the emergence of tardive dyskinesia. Monitoring of QT interval is also important with serial electrocardiograms. Overall, dopaminergic antagonists cause the more severe complication and therefore should be used cautiously.

Patients with medically refractory tics may be considered for deep brain stimulation procedure. However, the role of surgical therapy has not been determined yet, and this approach remains experimental.

Bibliography

Ackermans L, Duits A, van der Linden C, et al. Double-blind clinical trial of thalamic stimulation in patients with Tourette syndrome. Brain. 2011;134:832–44.

Alsene KM, Rajbhandari AK, Ramaker MJ, Bakshi VP. Discrete forebrain neuronal networks supporting noradrenergic regulation of sensorimotor gating. Neuropsychopharmacology. 2011;36:1003–14.

Bäumer T, Thomalla G, Kroeger J, et al. Interhemispheric motor networks are abnormal in patients with Gilles de la Tourette syndrome. Mov Disord. 2010;25:2828–37.

Bernabei M, Andreoni G, Mendez Garcia MO, et al. Automatic detection of tic activity in the Tourette Syndrome. Conf Proc IEEE Eng Med Biol Soc. 2010;2010:422–5.

Bloch M, State M, Pittenger C. Recent advances in Tourette syndrome. Curr Opin Neurol. 2011;24:119–25.

Bos-Veneman NG, Olieman R, Tobiasova Z, et al. Altered immunoglobulin profiles in children with Tourette syndrome. Brain Behav Immun. 2011;25:532–8.

Cath DC, Hedderly T, Ludolph AG, ESSTS Guidelines Group, et al. European clinical guidelines for Tourette syndrome and other tic disorders. Part I: assessment. Eur Child Adolesc Psychiatry. 2011;20:155–71.

Cavanna AE, Ali F, Rickards H. Paligraphia and written jocularity in Gilles de la Tourette syndrome. Mov Disord. 2011a;26:930–1.

Cavanna AE, Eddy CM, Mitchell R, et al. An approach to deep brain stimulation for severe treatment-refractory Tourette syndrome: the UK perspective. Br J Neurosurg. 2011b;25:38–44.

Copur M, Hergüner S, Arpaci B. Tolerability of quetiapine in children and adolescents with Tourette's syndrome. Int J Clin Pharmacol Ther. 2011;49:177–8.

Dávila G, Berthier ML, Kulisevsky J. Jurado Chacón S Suicide and attempted suicide in Tourette's syndrome: a case series with literature review. J Clin Psychiatry. 2010;71:1401–2.

Debes NM, Hansen A, Skov L, Larsson H. A functional magnetic resonance imaging study of a large clinical cohort of children with Tourette syndrome. J Child Neurol. 2011;26:560–9.

Dehning S, Feddersen B, Mehrkens JH, Müller N. Long-term results of electroconvulsive therapy in severe Gilles de la Tourette syndrome. J ECT. 2011;27:145–7.

Dhossche DM, Reti IM, Shettar SM, Wachtel LE. Tics as signs of catatonia: electroconvulsive therapy response in 2 men. J ECT. 2010;26:266–9.

Draganski B, Martino D, Cavanna AE, et al. Multispectral brain morphometry in Tourette syndrome persisting into adulthood. Brain. 2010;133:3661–75.

Du JC, Chiu TF, Lee KM, et al. Tourette syndrome in children: an updated review. Pediatr Neonatol. 2010;51:255–64.

Eapen V, Robertson MM, Alsobrook JP, et al. Obsessive compulsive symptoms in Gilles de la Tourette syndrome and obsessive compulsive disorder; difference by diagnosis and family history. Am J Med Genet. 1997;74:432–8.

Eddy CM, Cavanna AE, Gulisano M, et al. Clinical correlates of quality of life in Tourette syndrome. Mov Disord. 2011a;26:735–8.

Eddy CM, Rickards HE, Cavanna AE. Treatment strategies for tics in Tourette syndrome. Ther Adv Neurol Disord. 2011b;4:25–45.

Evans JG. Psychogenic pseudo-Tourette syndrome: one of Dr Johnson's maladies? J R Soc Med. 2010;103:500–2.

Freeman RD, Fast DK, Burd I, et al. Tourette Syndrome International Database Consortium. An international perspective on Tourette Syndrome: selected findings from 3,500 individuals in 22 countries. Dev Med Child Neurol. 2000;42:436–47.

Goetz CG, Pappert EJ. Textbook of clinical neurology. 2nd ed. Philadelphia: Saunders; 1999.

Hariz MI, Robertson MM. Gilles de la Tourette syndrome and deep brain stimulation. Eur J Neurosci. 2010;32:1128–34.

Jackson SR, Parkinson A, Jung J, et al. Compensatory neural reorganization in Tourette syndrome. Curr Biol. 2011;21:580–5.

Jankovic J. Phenomenology and classification of tics. Neurol Clin North Am. 1997;15:267–75.

Jankovic J. Tourette's syndrome. N Engl J Med. 2001;345:1184–92.

Jankovic J, Kurlan R. Tourette syndrome: evolving concepts. Mov Disord. 2011;26:1149–56.

Jankovic J, Tolosa E. Parkinson's disease and movement disorder. 5th ed. Philadelphia: Lippincott Williams & Wilkins; 2007.

Jankovic J, Mink J, Hollenbeck P, editors. Tourette's syndrome, Advances in neurology. Philadelphia: Lippincott Williams & Wilkins; 2006. p. 61–8.

Kantini E, Cassaday HJ, Hollis C, Jackson GM. The Normal Inhibition of Associations is Impaired by Clonidine in Tourette Syndrome. J Can Acad Child Adolesc Psychiatry. 2011;20:96–106.

Kompoliti K. The metabolic landscape of Tourette syndrome: learning to view the elephant as an elephant. Neurology. 2011;76:938–9.

Kurlan R. Clinical practice. Tourette's Syndrome. N Engl J Med. 2010;363:2332–8.

Kwak C, Dat Vuong K, Jankovic J. Premonitory sensory phenomenon in Tourette's syndrome. Mov Disord. 2003;18:1530–3.

Kwon HJ, Lim WS, Lim MH, et al. 1-Hz low frequency repetitive transcranial magnetic stimulation in children with Tourette's syndrome. Neurosci Lett. 2011;29(492):1–4.

Leckman JF, King RA, Gilbert DL, et al. Streptococcal upper respiratory tract infections and exacerbations of tic and obsessive-compulsive symptoms: a prospective longitudinal study. J Am Acad Child Adolesc Psychiatry. 2011;50:108–18.

Mack H, Fullana MA, Russell AJ, Mataix-Cols D, Nakatani E, Heyman I. Obsessions and compulsions in children with Asperger's syndrome or high-functioning autism: a case–control study. Aust N Z J Psychiatry. 2010;44:1082–8.

Maggio F, Pasciuto T, Paffi A, Apollonio F, Parazzini M, Ravazzani P, d'Inzeo G. Micro vs macro electrode DBS stimulation: a dosimetric study. Conf Proc IEEE Eng Med Biol Soc. 2010;2010:2057–60.

Martins GJ, Shahrokh M, Powell EM. Genetic disruption of Met signaling impairs GABAergic striatal development and cognition. Neuroscience. 2011;176:199–209.

Mathews CA, Grados MA. Familiality of Tourette syndrome, obsessive-compulsive disorder, and attention-deficit/hyperactivity disorder: heritability analysis in a large sib-pair sample. J Am Acad Child Adolesc Psychiatry. 2011;50:46–54.

Moll GH, Heinrich H, Troo GE, et al. Children with comorbid attention-deficit-hyperactivity disorder and tic disorder. Neurology. 2000;54:142–7.

Müller-Vahl KR, Cath DC, Cavanna AE, et al. ESSTS Guidelines Group. European clinical guidelines for Tourette syndrome and other tic disorders. Part IV: deep brain stimulation. Eur Child Adolesc Psychiatry. 2011;20:209–17.

Olfson M, Crystal S, Gerhard T, et al. Patterns and correlates of tic disorder diagnoses in privately and publicly insured youth. J Am Acad Child Adolesc Psychiatry. 2011;50:119–31.

Pourfar M, Feigin A, Tang CC, et al. Abnormal metabolic brain networks in Tourette syndrome. Neurology. 2011;76:944–52.

Rajapakse T, Pringsheim T. Pharmacotherapeutics of Tourette syndrome and stereotypies in autism. Semin Pediatr Neurol. 2010;17:254–60.

Ramirez-Bermudez J, Perez-Rincon H. A proper name for chronic tic disorder. Am J Psychiatry. 2010;167:1279.

Ray LW, Koller WC. Movement disorders, neurologic principles and practice. 2nd ed. New York: McGraw-Hill; 1997.

Rizzo R, Gulisano M, Calì PV, Curatolo P. ADHD and epilepsy in children with Tourette syndrome: a triple comorbidity? Acta Paediatr. 2010;99:1894–6.

Robertson MM. Tourette syndrome, associated conditions, and the complexities of treatment. Brain. 2000;123:425–62.

Roessner V, Plessen KJ, Rothenberger A, et al. ESSTS Guidelines Group. European clinical guidelines for Tourette syndrome and other tic disorders. Part II: pharmacological treatment. Eur Child Adolesc Psychiatry. 2011a;20:173–96.

Roessner V, Rothenberger A, Rickards H, Hoekstra PJ. European clinical guidelines for Tourette syndrome and other tic disorders. Eur Child Adolesc Psychiatry. 2011b;20:153–4.

Rolands LP, editor. Merritt's textbook of neurology. 10th ed. New York: Lippincott Williams & Wilkins; 2000.

Servello D, Sassi M, Gaeta M, Ricci C, Porta M. Tourette syndrome (TS) bears a higher rate of inflammatory complications at the implanted hardware in deep brain stimulation (DBS). Acta Neurochir (Wien). 2011;153:629–32.

Singer HS. Current issues in Tourette syndrome. Mov Disord. 2000;15:1051–63.

Singer HS. Tourette's syndrome: from behaviour to biology. Lancet Neurol. 2005;4:149–59.

Singer HS. Tourette syndrome and other tic disorders. Handb Clin Neurol. 2011;100:641–57.

State MW. The genetics of Tourette disorder. Curr Opin Genet Dev. 2011;21:302–9.

Sukhodolsky DG, Landeros-Weisenberger A, Scahill L, Leckman JF, Schultz RT. Neuropsychological functioning in children with Tourette syndrome with and without attention-deficit/hyperactivity disorder. J Am Acad Child Adolesc Psychiatry. 2010;49:1155–64.

Sundaram SK, Huq AM, Sun Z, et al. Exome sequencing of a pedigree with Tourette syndrome or chronic tic disorder. Ann Neurol. 2011;69:901–4.

Sutherland Owens AN, Miguel EC, Swerdlow NR. Sensory gating scales and premonitory urges in Tourette syndrome. ScientificWorldJournal. 2011;11:736–41.

Termine C, Selvini C, Balottin U, Luoni C, Eddy CM, Cavanna AE. Self-, parent-, and teacher-reported behavioral symptoms in youngsters with Tourette syndrome: a case–control study. Eur J Paediatr Neurol. 2011;15:95–100.

The Tourette's Syndrome Classification Study Group. Definitions and classification of tic disorders. Arch Neurol. 1993;50:1013–6.

Verdellen C, van de Griendt J, Hartmann A, Murphy T, ESSTS Guidelines Group. European clinical guidelines for Tourette syndrome and other tic disorders. Part III: behavioural and psychosocial interventions. Eur Child Adolesc Psychiatry. 2011;20:197–207.

Walusinski O. Keeping the fire burning: Georges Gilles de la Tourette, Paul Richer, Charles Féré and Alfred Binet. Front Neurol Neurosci. 2011;29:71–90.

Walusinski O, Bogousslavsky J. Georges Gilles de la Tourette (1857–1904). J Neurol. 2011;258:166–7.

Werner CJ, Stöcker T, Kellermann T, et al. Altered amygdala functional connectivity in adult Tourette's syndrome. Eur Arch Psychiatry Clin Neurosci. 2010;260 Suppl 2:S95–9.

Worbe Y, Gerardin E, Hartmann A, et al. Distinct structural changes underpin clinical phenotypes in patients with Gilles de la Tourette syndrome. Brain. 2010;133:3649–60.

Yaltho TC, Jankovic J, Lotze T. The association of Tourette syndrome and dopa-responsive dystonia. Mov Disord. 2011;26:359–60.

Zou LP, Wang Y, Zhang LP, et al. Tourette syndrome and excitatory substances: is there a connection? Childs Nerv Syst. 2011;27:793–802.

Chapter 5
Myoclonus

Abstract Myoclonus is characterized by brief involuntary muscle jerks due to concise electromyographic bursts of 10–50 ms. Abnormal movements can be induced by both positive muscle contractions or negative symptoms with brief lapses of muscle contractions. This chapter reviews main clinical characteristics of myoclonus and its most common causes. We describe characteristic phenotypic features of myoclonus, classification based on clinical presentation and pathophysiology of myoclonus, and therapeutic options to control this abnormal movement.

Keywords Myoclonus • Asterixis • Muscle contraction • Opsoclonus-myoclonus • Corticobasal degeneration

Myoclonus refers to brief, lightning-like involuntary muscle jerks due to concise electromyographic bursts of 10–50 ms. These brief lightning-like jerks are rarely more than 100 ms in duration, and affect the extremities, face, and the trunk. The jerks are generally caused by positive muscle contractions, but can also be a result of sudden brief lapses of contraction, as seen in *asterixis*.

A.Q. Rana, P. Hedera, *Differential Diagnosis of Movement Disorders in Clinical Practice*, DOI 10.1007/978-3-319-01607-8_5,
© Springer International Publishing Switzerland 2014

5.1   Classification

Myoclonus can be classified by site of origin, clinical features, response to stimulus, and etiology.

However, myoclonus can also be classified according to physiology which helps in identifying the underlying process and thus treatment.

5.1.1   Classification Based upon Site of Origin

Cortical Myoclonus

Cortical myoclonus is the most common form of myoclonus. It arises from the sensorimotor cortex and is generally arrhythmic. Focal or multifocal jerks may also be apparent due to spontaneity or induction by reflex or action. Following are some of the common conditions in which cortical myoclonus may be seen:

1. Progressive myoclonic epilepsies include Unverricht-Lundborg disease, Lafora disease, MERRF, DRPLA, familial adult myoclonic epilepsy, idiopathic progressive myoclonic epilepsy, Angelman syndrome, and celiac disease.
2. Encephalopathies caused by HIV metabolic or toxic conditions.
3. Alzheimer's disease.
4. Gaucher's disease.
5. Creutzfeldt-Jakob disease.

Subcortical Myoclonus

Subcortical myoclonus is thought to be caused by metabolic and hypoxic dysfunction such as hepatic or renal failure. The brainstem and thalamus are usually involved in this type of myoclonus, which normally manifests itself as stimulus sensitive and generalized.

Spinal Myoclonus

Spinal myoclonus is usually associated with the presence of a focal lesion and is only rarely idiopathic. The lesion may compress the spinal cord or may have minimal mass effect. It is usually divided into two types, i.e., segmental spinal myoclonus and propriospinal myoclonus. Segmental spinal myoclonus may be rhythmic in nature and non-stimulus sensitive. In propriospinal myoclonus, the lesion is normally at the thoracic level and movements are more widespread than those observed in segmental spinal myoclonus. Propriospinal myoclonus may lead to episodic flexion of trunk with myoclonus. As mentioned above, the typical cause of spinal myoclonus is the presence of a focal spinal lesion such as trauma, syringomyelia, multiple sclerosis, an infection (e.g., herpes zoster, Lyme's disease, or HIV), or ischemic myelopathy. Imaging of spinal cord, EMG as well as somatosensory evoke potentials (SSEP) may be helpful in localizing the site of pathology. Spinal myoclonus may cause significant interference in mobility in some cases.

Peripheral Myoclonus

The most frequently observed peripheral myoclonus is hemifacial spasm, which is idiopathic in nature and is believed to be caused by compression of the facial nerve. Hemifacial spasm is unilateral in most of the cases and is characterized by intermittent clonic contractions of the muscles of face.

Some of the studies have suggested that lesions of the peripheral nerves may change inhibitory spinal interneurons and sensory input.

5.1.2   Classification Based upon Clinical Features

Clinically, myoclonus can be classified by many different ways, e.g., site of involvement, amplitude of movements, frequency of movements, present with action, intended movements, or at rest. The jerks associated with myoclonus may occur repeatedly or individually. They may be generalized, focal, multifocal, or segmental.

1. *Generalized myoclonus* involves synchronous jerks of one or more major muscle groups.
2. *Focal myoclonus* involves movements restricted to defined body parts; most common is spinal myoclonus, propriospinal myoclonus, arm myoclonus, and hemifacial spasm.

3. *Multifocal myoclonus* involves two or more nonadjacent areas of the body.
4. *Segmental myoclonus* involves adjacent areas of the body usually due to trauma and inflammation or tumor.

The amplitude of the jerks observed in myoclonus ranges from mild contractions that do not move a joint to more severe larger contractions that move the head, limbs, or trunk. Myoclonic jerks vary in frequency from occasional isolated events to multiple episodes which may appear almost continuously. They may arise with indented movements, at rest, or with action. Myoclonic jerks may be stimulus sensitive, and can be aggravated by visual threat, noise, pinprick, movement, or light. Myoclonic jerks may occur sporadically and unpredictably. Some of the myoclonic jerks may occur in bursts of oscillations, whereas others are very intermittent, as in palatal myoclonus. In such a case, the jerks may resemble tremor.

Myoclonus that originates from the cerebral cortex is termed *cortical myoclonus* and is usually reflex induced and focal. The cortical source of myoclonus can be established by the observation of spikes in the electroencephalogram associated with electromyographic correlated jerks.

Myoclonus that originates from the brainstem can be either segmental (e.g., *oculo-palatal-pharyngeal myoclonus*) or generalized (e.g., reticular myoclonus). Palatal myoclonus is rhythmical (around 2 Hz) and can be classified as primary or secondary. Secondary palatal myoclonus is more common and is caused by a lesion within the Guillain-Mollaret triangle encompassing the red nucleus, inferior olivary nuclei, and dentate. This causes an interruption of the dentatoolivary pathway, leading to the denervation of the olives, which can become hypertrophic. Multiple sclerosis and vascular lesions are frequent causes of secondary palatal myoclonus which may persist during sleep.

Myoclonus originating from the spinal cord consists of two clinical forms. *Propriospinal myoclonus* causes truncal flexion along with jerks, usually caused by a stimulus. The other clinical form of myoclonus originating from the spinal cord is *spinal segmental myoclonus*, which is rhythmic and may also occur during sleep. In propriospinal myoclonus, the first muscles to be activated are generally from the thoracic cord, with slow downward and upward spread. Myoclonic jerks can sometimes occur from a peripheral nerve, spinal root, or plexus.

Rasmussen encephalitis is a disorder of childhood or adolescence characterized by unilateral focal seizures, including epilepsia partialis continua and a progressive hemiplegia.

5.1.3 Classification Based upon Provocative Factors

Myoclonic movement can be classified based on response to movements or certain stimuli. The movements can be either spontaneous, in which no stimulus is needed to induce it, or it may appear in response to stimulus. Common causes of spontaneous myoclonus are metabolic encephalopathies of Creutzfeldt-Jakob disease.

Reflex myoclonus occurs in response to verbal, somesthetic, or auditory stimulus. Hyperekplexia is an exaggerated startle reflex which can be idiopathic or genetic in terms of etiology. Action myoclonus is very disabling as it causes disruption of volitional movements that are associated with provocative factors.

5.1.4 Classification Based upon Etiology

Myoclonus can be classified into the following etiologic categories:

1. Physiologic myoclonus
2. Essential myoclonus
3. Epileptic myoclonus
4. Symptomatic myoclonus

Physiologic myoclonus is a normal phenomenon with no associated disability. Hypnic jerks, benign sleep myoclonus of infancy generally occurring in the immediate postpartum period, and hiccoughs are some of the examples of physiologic myoclonus.

Essential myoclonus is idiopathic, without any progressive course, and is not linked with other neurologic conditions. It is generally multifocal in distribution and coexists with features of dystonia in some patients. Some patients may have a positive family history.

Epileptic myoclonus occurs in patients with generalized convulsions but patients also have myoclonus. Most patients have cognitive dysfunction such as seen in Lafora disease and neuronal ceroid-lipofuscinosis.

Symptomatic myoclonus occurs as part of an encephalopathic process due to many different neurological conditions such as dementias, spinocerebellar degenerations, storage diseases, focal brain damage, and toxic, infectious, metabolic, and physical encephalopathies. Whipple disease is an infectious condition which has facial myoclonus known as oculofacial-masticatory myorhythmia. Serotonin syndrome is a type of toxic encephalopathy and is caused by medications that produce extreme serotonergic stimulation.

5.2   Investigations

Serum glucose levels, liver function tests, electrolytes, and screening studies for antibodies, drugs, and toxins may be helpful in assessment of different causes of myoclonus. Imaging studies such as MRI of the brain may be required in some cases.

Electromyography may help to localize the site of pathology in spinal myoclonus, and electroencephalography is used to assess the cortical involvement in myoclonus. Genetic testing can also be done where a familial cause, such as dentatorubral-pallidoluysian atrophy, and myoclonic epilepsy are suspected.

5.3   Causes

5.3.1   *Opsoclounus Myoclonus Syndrome*

Opsoclonus-myoclonus syndrome or polyminimyoclonus is a rare type of myoclonic syndrome in which the myoclonic jerks are of minimal amplitude. Patients have irregular, chaotic, and spontaneous saccadic movements of eyes; hence, the term "dancing eyes," or opsoclonus, is used to describe the ocular movements. Although initially described in children in association with a neuroblastoma, it is also observed in adults in postviral or paraneoplastic syndrome.

5.3.2   Exaggerated Startle Syndromes

Patients with exaggerated startle syndromes present with abnormal myoclonic movements in response to unexpected tactile, visual, or auditory stimuli. These movements are believed to originate from the brainstem. Examples of such stimuli are a blink, flexion and abduction of the arms, contraction of the face, and flexion of the trunk and neck.

5.3.3   Hyperekplexia

Hyperekplexia is a type of primary myoclonus and is referred to as *stiff baby syndrome* when the onset is in childhood. It is inherited in an autosomal dominant fashion with mutation on chromosome 5q. This chromosome is responsible for coding the α_1 subunit of the inhibitory glycine receptor. The extended tonic spasms occur when the child is handled which may result in apnea causing death in some cases. These episodes of spasm and myoclonus are managed with anticonvulsants such as valproic acid and clonazepam, as well as with the serotonin precursor 5-hydroxytryptophan. Treatment may involve use of many medications including primidone, clonazepam, piracetam, and sodium valproate.

5.3.4   Corticobasal Degeneration

Patients with corticobasal degeneration may have stimulus-sensitive myoclonus. Corticobasal degeneration is a rare condition, although the exact incidence and prevalence is unknown. Estimated incidence is 0.60–0.90 cases per 100,000 populations. Average survival rate is of 7–8 years, and it is a sporadic disorder.

The usual age of onset is in the sixth to eighth decade of life. Patients have combination of symptoms including clumsiness, stiffness, sensory impairment, and jerkiness usually involving one arm. There is rigidity, bradykinesia, and apraxia of the involved limb and there may not be any significant intellectual impairment initially. Patients display a minimal response to L-dopa.

Asymmetry of the involved limb is characteristic of this disorder. In a significant minority of CBD patients, there is a rigid dystonic arm with some fingers extended and others forcibly flexed. The dystonic arm may jerk irregularly due to action-induced and stimulus-sensitive reflex myoclonus. However, corticobasal degeneration does not feature the distinctive resting tremor of Parkinson's disease.

One half of all corticobasal degeneration patients may have the alien limb phenomena. In the dominant hand, ALP is distinguished by a strong grasp reflex and an intractable compulsion to reach for and manipulate objects. An alien limb phenomenon is not specific for corticobasal degeneration however and may also be seen in cases of Alzheimer's and Creutzfeldt-Jakob disease.

Numbness in corticobasal degeneration may result from sensory extinction, astereognosis, agraphesthesia, and impaired 2-point discrimination. Signs of corticospinal tract dysfunction (extensor plantar responses and exaggerated deep tendon reflexes), frontal release signs (grasp) and bulbar dysfunction, and visual inattention are common in the later courses of corticobasal degeneration. Communication is often impaired by dysarthria, while dysphagia with resulting aspiration pneumonia is a major cause of mortality and morbidity.

Corticobasal degeneration frequently presents with the dysexecutive phenotype of frontal dementia. Corticobasal degeneration should be suspected when patients are afflicted with dementia involving limited attention/concentration, dysphagia, executive dysfunction, behavioral changes, urinary incontinence, and bilateral motor signs (such as parkinsonism) and pyramidal signs.

MRI may show asymmetric pericentral cortical atrophy in majority of corticobasal degeneration patients. There is a mild frontoparietal cortical atrophy in most of the cases. It is characterized by abnormal deposition of the tau protein; this tau accumulation generally occurs in the basal ganglia and cerebral cortex. Diagnosis of corticobasal degeneration is based on history and physical examination.

There currently exists no treatment for delaying or preventing the onset of corticobasal degeneration; symptomatic therapy is generally ineffectual. Corticobasal degeneration patients exhibit minimal response to L-dopa. Clonazepam may reduce myoclonus, while botulinum toxin injections may relieve limb dystonia. Pharmacological drugs such as baclofen, steroids, anticholinergics, and anticonvulsants are not particularly useful as treatments for corticobasal degeneration. In addition to drug therapy, physical therapy for gait disturbances may prevent falls. Occupational therapy may minimize the impact of disabilities. A weighted glove may be placed on the less affected limb to promote the use of the affected hand and may provide some benefit to the patients with rigid stiff arm. Speech therapy for dysarthria, dietitian assessment for dysphagia, and use of percutaneous gastrostomy may be required in the course of corticobasal degeneration.

Bibliography

Belcastro V, Arnaboldi M, Taborelli A, Prontera P. Induction of epileptic negative myoclonus by addition of lacosamide to carbamazepine. Epilepsy Behav. 2011;20:589–90.

Beukers RJ, Foncke EM, van der Meer JN, Veltman DJ, Tijssen MA. Functional magnetic resonance imaging evidence of incomplete maternal imprinting in myoclonus-dystonia. Arch Neurol. 2011;68:802–5.

Brackmann FA, Kiefer A, Agaimy A, Gencik M, Trollmann R. Rapidly progressive phenotype of Lafora disease associated with a novel NHLRC1 mutation. Pediatr Neurol. 2011;44:475–7.

Brown P. The startle syndrome. Mov Disord. 2002;17 Suppl 2:579–82.

Canafoglia L, Franceschetti S, Uziel G, et al. Characterization of severe action myoclonus in sialidoses. Epilepsy Res. 2011;94:86–93.

Carroll E, Sanchez-Ramos J. Hyperkinetic movement disorders associated with HIV and other viral infections. Handb Clin Neurol. 2011; 100:323–34.

Caveness JN, Brown P. Myoclonus: current concepts and recent advances. Lancet Neurol. 2004;3:598–607.

Caviness JN, Truong DD. Myoclonus. Handb Clin Neurol. 2011;100:399–420.

De Falco FS, Striano P, de Falso A, et al. Benign adult familial myoclonic epilepsy: genetic heterogeneity and allelism with ADCME. Neurology. 2003;60:1381–5.

Dibbens LM, Karakis I, Bayly MA, Costello DJ, Cole AJ, Berkovic SF. Mutation of SCARB2 in a patient with progressive myoclonus epilepsy and demyelinating peripheral neuropathy. Arch Neurol. 2011; 68:812–3.

Dressler D. Nonprimary dystonias. Handb Clin Neurol. 2011;100:513–38.

Floeter MK, Andermann F, Andermann E, et al. Physiological studies of spinal inhibitory pathways in patients with hereditary hyperekplexia. Neurology. 1996;46:766–72.

Frauscher B, Kunz A, Brandauer E, Ulmer H, Poewe W, Högl B. Fragmentary myoclonus in sleep revisited: a polysomnographic study in 62 patients. Sleep Med. 2011;12:410–5.

Gaig C, Valldeoriola F, Gelpi E, et al. Rapidly progressive diffuse Lewy body disease. Mov Disord. 2011;26:1316–23.

Gershanik OS, Gómez Arévalo GJ. Typical and atypical neuroleptics. Handb Clin Neurol. 2011;100:579–99.

Goetz CG, Pappert EJ. Textbook of clinical neurology. 2nd ed. Philadelphia: Saunders; 1999.

Gordon MF. Toxin and drug induced myoclonus. Adv Neurol. 2002;89:49–76.

Groen J, van Rootselaar AF, van der Salm SM, Bloem BR, Tijssen M. A new familial syndrome with dystonia and lower limb action myoclonus. Mov Disord. 2011;26:896–900.

Hajdu CH, Lefkowitch JH. Adult polyglucosan body disease: a rare presentation with chronic liver disease and ground-glass hepatocellular inclusions. Semin Liver Dis. 2011;31:223–9.

Hallet M, Chadwick D, Marsden CD. Cortical reflex myoclonus. Neurology. 1979;29:1107–25.

Hanajima R, Terao Y, Nakatani-Enomoto S, et al. Triad stimulation frequency for cortical facilitation in cortical myoclonus. Mov Disord. 2011; 26:685–90.

Haverkaemper S, Marquardt T, Hausser I, et al. Congenital ichthyosis in severe type II Gaucher disease with a homozygous null mutation. Neonatology. 2011;100:194–7.

Ishibashi T, Ishibashi S, Uchida T, Nakazawa K, Makita K. Reversible cerebral vasoconstriction syndrome with limb myoclonus following intravenous administration of methylergometrine. J Anesth. 2011;25:405–8.

Jankovic J, Tolosa E. Parkinson's disease and movement disorder. 5th ed. Philadelphia: Lippincott Williams & Wilkins; 2007.

Jimenez-Jimenez FJ, Puertas I, De Toledo-Heras M. Drug induced myoclonus: frequency, mechanisms and management. CNS Drugs. 2004; 8:93–104.

Kawarai T, Tsuda R, Taniguchi K, et al. Spinal myoclonus resulting from intrathecal administration of human neural stem cells. Mov Disord. 2011;26:1358–60.

Khan WU, Staios G, Rana AQ. Paroxysmal kinesigenic dyskinesia in a mother and daughter. Acta Neurol Belg. 2010;110:201–2.

Kojovic M, Cordivari C, Bhatia K. Myoclonic disorders: a practical approach for diagnosis and treatment. Ther Adv Neurol Disord. 2011;4: 47–462.

Kouri N, Whitwell JL, Josephs KA, Rademakers R, Dickson DW. Corticobasal degeneration: a pathologically distinct 4R tauopathy. Nat Rev Neurol. 2011;7:263–72.

Kowarik MC, Langer S, Keri C, Hemmer B, Oexle K, Winkelmann J. Myoclonus-dystonia in 18p deletion syndrome. Mov Disord. 2011;26: 560–1.

Mima T, Nagamine T, Nishitani N, et al. Cortical myoclonus: sensorimotor herexcitability. Neurology. 1998;50:933–42.

Nardocci N. Myoclonus-dystonia syndrome. Handb Clin Neurol. 2011;100: 563–75.

Nunes JC, Bruscato AM, Walz R, Lin K. Opsoclonus-myoclonus syndrome associated with Mycoplasma pneumoniae infection in an elderly patient. J Neurol Sci. 2011;305:147–8.

O'Riordan S, Ozelius LJ, De Carvalho Aguiar P, et al. Inherited myoclonus-dystonia and epilepsy. Further evidence of an association? Mov Disord. 2004;19:1456–9.

Perlman SL. Spinocerebellar degenerations. Handb Clin Neurol. 2011;100: 113–40.

Pfeffer G, Abegg M, Vertinsky AT, Ceccherini I, Caroli F, Barton JJ. The ocular motor features of adult-onset alexander disease: a case and review of the literature. J Neuroophthalmol. 2011;31:155–9.

Polajnar M, Zerovnik E. Impaired autophagy: a link between neurodegenerative diseases and progressive myoclonus epilepsies. Trends Mol Med. 2011;17:293–300.

Ray LW, Koller WC. Movement disorders, neurologic principles and practice. 2nd ed. New York: McGraw-Hill; 1997.

Rolands LP, editor. Merritt's textbook of neurology. 10th ed. New York: Lippincott Williams & Wilkins; 2000.

Sahu JK, Prasad K. The opsoclonus-myoclonus syndrome. Pract Neurol. 2011;11:160–6.

Shibasaki H, Thompson PD. Milestones in myoclonus. Mov Disord. 2011; 26:1142–8.

Tagliabracci VS, Heiss C, Karthik C, et al. Phosphate incorporation during glycogen synthesis and Lafora disease. Cell Metab. 2011;13: 274–82.

Tremolizzo L, Fermi S, Fusco ML, et al. Generalized action myoclonus associated with escitalopram in a patient with mixed dementia. J Clin Psychopharmacol. 2011;31:394–5.

Umeda Y, Matsuda H, Sadamori H, et al. Leukoencephalopathy syndrome after living-donor liver transplantation. Exp Clin Transplant. 2011;9:139–44.

van Gaalen J, Giunti P, van de Warrenburg BP. Movement disorders in spinocerebellar ataxias. Mov Disord. 2011;26:792–800.

Van Rootselaar A, Aronica E, Jansen Steur ENH, et al. Familial cortical tremor with epilepsy and cerebellar pathological findings. Mov Disord. 2004;19:213–7.

Vernia S, Heredia M, Criado O, et al. Laforin, a dual specificity phosphatase involved in Lafora disease, regulates insulin response and whole-body energy balance in mice. Hum Mol Genet. 2011;20: 2571–84.

Yamada K, Sakurama T, Soyama N, Kuratsu J. Gpi pallidal stimulation for Lance-Adams syndrome. Neurology. 2011;76:1270–2.

Zamponi N, Passamonti C, Luzi M, Trignani R, Regnicolo L, Scarpelli M. Fourth ventricle hamartoma presenting with progressive myoclonus and hemifacial spasms: case report and review of literature. Childs Nerv Syst. 2011;27:1001–5.

Zesiewicz TA, Sullivan KL. Drug-induced hyperkinetic movement disorders by nonneuroleptic agents. Handb Clin Neurol. 2011;100: 347–63.

Index

A.Q. Rana, P. Hedera, *Differential Diagnosis of Movement*
Disorders in Clinical Practice, DOI 10.1007/978-3-319-01607-8,
© Springer International Publishing Switzerland 2014